How to Develop Drug

How to Develop Drug Products

A Sequential Approach

Murat Kulahci
Anil Menon

Datanumerix LLC

Publisher's Cataloging-in-Publication data
Names: Kulahci, Murat, author. | Menon, Anil B., author.
Title: How to develop drug products: a sequential approach /
Murat Kulahci and Anil Menon.
Description: Includes bibliographical references. | Morrisville,
NC: Datanumerix LLC, 2023.
Identifiers: LCCN: 2022920440 | ISBN: 9798987108611
Subjects: LCSH Drug development. | Pharmaceutical technology. |
Experimental design. | BISAC TECHNOLOGY & ENGINEERING /
Pharmaceutical | MATHEMATICS / Statistics
Classification: LCC RM301.25 .K85 2023 | DDC 615.19–dc23

Published by Datanumerix LLC. P O Box 1026, Morrisville,
NC 27560.

Designed and typeset by 16LEAVES
www.16leaves.com

To the memory of
Professor Søren Bisgaard: machinist, engineer, statistician, and an exceptional educator.

All the factors are seldom known, and sometimes even the response and the objective are unknown. Thus, one should proceed step by step with relatively small experiments and use what is learned from previous experiments to plan the next.

—Søren Bisgaard, 1993

Contents

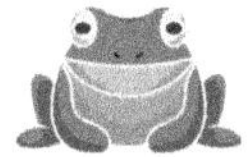

A Word From the Authors

Thank you for starting from the beginning. This book is for formulators and managers who want an adaptive approach to developing drug products. Drug product development results from an investigation that involves a sequence of experiments. In this book we describe this journey, describing how each subset of experimental runs combined with subject matter knowledge helps drug developers decide what to do next.

Chapters 1 to 5 briefly introduce sequential experimentation, the drug product development stages, and experimental design using four experiments. One can understand these chapters as well as Chapter 10 without knowing experimental design details, just as you do not need to understand automotive technology to drive your car. The simple mnemonics on the inside, front, and back covers can be used as a quick checklist for experimental design thinking and analysis.

Chapter 6 introduces essential ideas in factorial and fractional factorial designs and their analysis. These designs are a staple of product development programs. Chapters 7 to 9 are practical case studies, and Chapter 10 summarizes lessons we have learned from our mistakes, including examples. We use numerical and graphical data analysis as well as our expertise to interpret the data and decide what to do next. We deliberately avoided giving comprehensive statistical analyses to keep the theme of encouraging design thinking

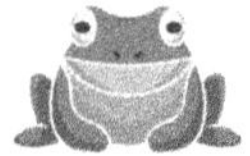

and sequential experimentation for developing pharmaceutical products. Please refer to the statistical analyses posted on datatodecision.org. The statistical and graphical analyses are done in R, an open-source software.

The chapters are brief, and the references provide material for going deeper into the topics. Blank cells in a data table are cells without any data. They do not represent missing or overlooked data.

An obvious caution: We can study every book, attend every tutorial, and calculate the ideal number of experimental trials nonstop. However, there is no substitute for hands-on experience in designing and analyzing experiments. This book can only provide a framework as you grapple with the subjective choices in designing an experiment, overcome challenges that will inevitably arise, and adapt when something goes wrong.

We hope that like us you find the journey ultimately rewarding, and that you enjoy experimenting despite the challenges you will face. We also hope and believe that this book can help you avoid pitfalls.

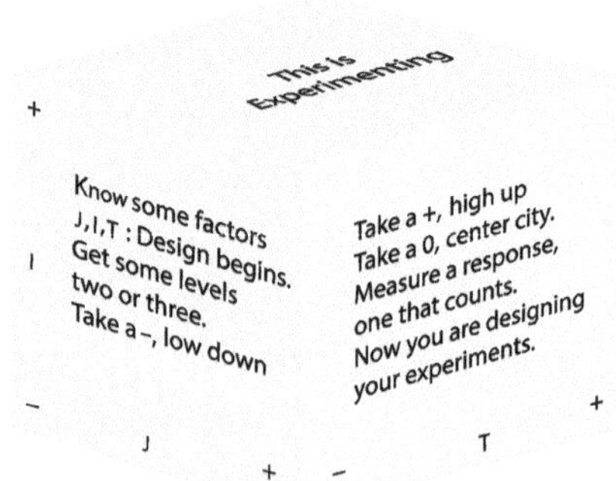

This Is
Experimenting
Know some factors
J, I, T : Design begins.
Get some levels
two or three.
Take a –, low down
Take a +, high up
Take a 0, center city.
Measure a response,
one that counts.
Now you are designing
your experiments.
+
I
–
J
+
–
T
+

1

Introduction

Physicist and philosopher Hermann von Helmholtz, who is known for developing the principle of conservation of energy, described his approach to scientific inquiry thus:

> I liken myself to a mountaineer who climbs slowly and laboriously without knowing the path, frequently having to turn around when they can't go any farther. They eventually arrive at their destination after stumbling into new pathways by accident and deliberate choices. But to their shame, they discover a royal way they may have been able to ascend—had they been clever enough to discover it at first. In my writing, I don't entertain the reader with my wanderings; instead, I describe the paved route they can follow to the top without exertion.

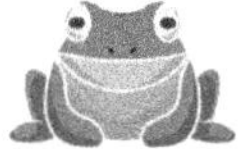

While von Helmholtz's slow and laborious climb created crucial insights, drug product development will benefit significantly if we use the "royal road." Statisticians, scientists, and technicians have outlined that route for product development: using the sequential experimental design[1] approach with subject matter knowledge. In this approach, product developers working in groups explore unfamiliar territory systematically, advancing step by step and drawing on the steps already taken in determining the next.

Multiple groups contribute subject matter knowledge, market needs, financial forecasts, regulatory guidance, technical know-how, training, experience, budgets, and opinions. Project goals shift direction over time, triggered by obstacles, unexpected results, or new organizational goals. Using a sequential experimental design approach makes it easier to adapt to these shifts and achieve a satisfactory outcome.

Product development is an interplay between ideas, goals, and experimentation. The development stage defines the scope and scale of experiments:

- Technical product development moves forward by the union of experimental data and subject matter knowledge. Association of the two streams flowing together dates to Galileo's understanding that the two methods, the empirical (experimental data) and the logical (subject matter knowledge), are meaningless alone. Experimenters move between experimenting, analyzing, and thinking about the results until they satisfice[2] a goal.

---

1 "Design," here, does not mean designing the dosage form (tablet, capsule), the drug delivery system, or the equipment. In experimentation, "design" refers to the act of determining a set of experiments.

2 Herbert A. Simon introduced *satisfice*, a portmanteau of satisfy and suffice, in his 1956 acceptance speech of the Nobel Prize in Economics. He observed that "decision makers can satisfice either by finding optimum solutions for a simplified world, or by finding satisfactory solutions for a more realistic world. Neither approach, in general, dominates the other, and both have continued to co-exist in the world of management science."

- Understanding the product development stages helps decide the experimental design, the number of experimental trials, people, budget, and time for a program. We use experimental design and testing at each stage of an idea, prototype, product, manufacture, or commercial supply.

Recall Helmholtz's mountain metaphor to understand the sequential design approach. We want to climb higher. We could take any route that looks promising, hoping for the best, but we may not get far or reach our destination before winter comes. Or we could use subject matter knowledge and experimental design to learn effectively (Figure 1.1) and decide *what to do next*. We start with an initial experiment. Based on the results, we may add more experiments, or replicate, followed by adding more factors, moving to a new location, or rescaling. Product development is an iterative process, which follows a trail often not predictable in advance.

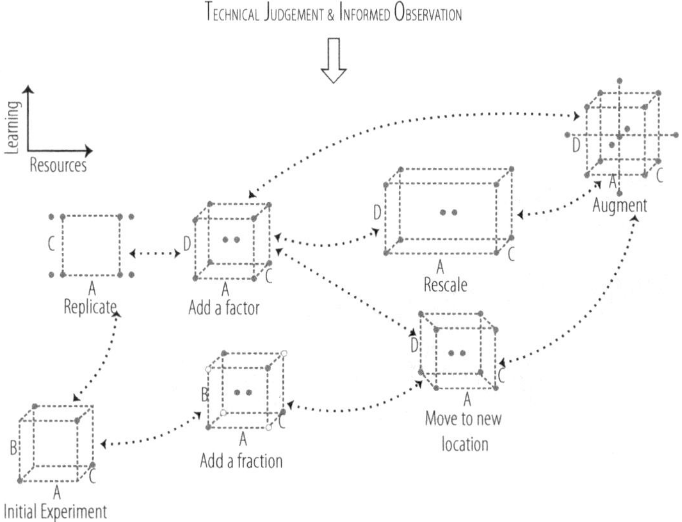

Figure 1.1: Alternatives for deciding the next set of experiments depending on the previous results. A, B, C, D represent factors such as pH, temperature, force, type, or percentage of an excipient we are studying.

NOTES

Hemholtz's quote from his remarks on his 70th birthday is translated and paraphrased from Helmhothz, H. V. (1892). *Ansprachen und Reden, gehalten bei der am 2. November 1891 zu Ehren von Hermann von Helmholtz veranstalteten Feier*, 54. Berlin: Hirschwald.

Kahl, R. ed. (1971). *Selected Writings of Hermann von Helmholtz*. Middletown, CT: Wesleyan University Press.

Kulahci, M. and Box, G.E.P. (2003). Catalysis of discovery and development in engineering and industry. *Quality Engineering* 15 (3): 513–517.

Meleshko, V.V. and Aref, H. (2007). A bibliography of vortex dynamics 1858–1956. *Advances in Applied Mechanics* 41: 197–292.

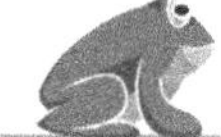

The mathematical subject of experimental design has many potential pitfalls. The experimenter might choose the wrong variables, explore the wrong region, or use inappropriate scaling. However, we adaptively arrive at a satisfactory solution because we know the subject matter and experiment sequentially. This sequential and iterative experimental approach acts as a corrective loop.

2

Why Run Experiments Sequentially?

The essence of sequential experimentation is a series of experiments each of which depends on what has gone on before.

— R. A. Fisher, 1952

Experimentation is a tool to develop products. Every experiment yields information. Early ideas or paths may not work out, and new ideas and trails may enter the investigation. The product features may change, and the goals may shift. We discover the route to the destination as we experiment, as each subset of experimental trials shapes future experimentation. The path to developing products is not straightforward. The experimenter adapts to the information and circumstances, then decides *what to do next.*

The late statistician-scientist George Box defined experimentation as a path to guided learning. The experimental design makes the course as efficient as possible and helps

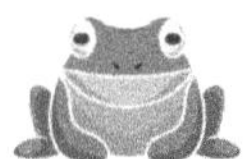

answer *what to do next.* At first sight, planning experiments appears arbitrary and uncertain. Teams must consider various questions during the planning phase:

1. Which technology (e.g., roller compaction, wet granulation) should we use?
2. Which factors (e.g., roll pressure, roll gap) in the chosen technology should we study?
3. Should we study factors independently, or do we take ratios?
4. Do we study the category or quantity of a factor? For example, is polymer type or polymer concentration necessary?
5. How do we choose the many possibilities in a category?
6. How many levels (e.g., two - or three-roll pressures) should we study?
7. Which responses (e.g., percentage of degradation, percentage dissolved) do we study?
8. What is the correct experimental scale? Which batch size?
9. How much time and critical raw material(s) are available?
10. Do we have the needed equipment, instrumentation, and measurement methods?
11. Can we schedule the required equipment in our laboratories or plant?
12. What if we fail in achieving our objective or ultimate goal?

These questions are subject to opinion and judgment, yet they can guide the successful development of products when we use iterative experiments and our subject matter knowledge. We do not complete one grand experiment when we know the least. Instead, we conduct a series of small experimental designs, analyzing, adapting, and getting new ideas as we move toward a goal. This flexible approach allows us to learn through periods of progress and stagnation. We use subject matter knowledge to guide our experiments to reach a satisfactory conclusion regardless of the starting point. George Box summarized the learning by experiment through repeated use of IDEAS (Idea, Design, Experiment, Analyze, Summarize):

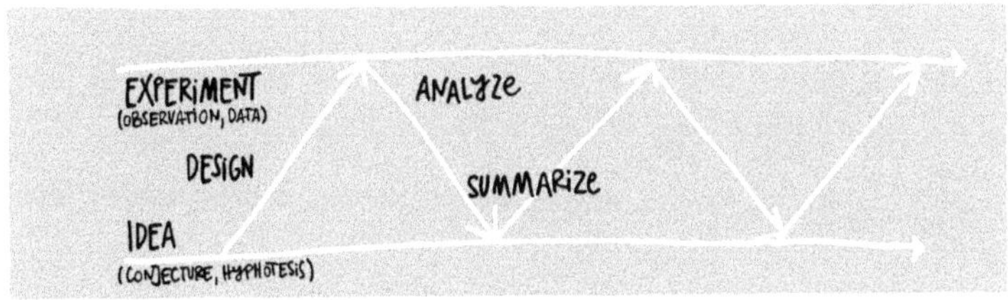

Learning by sequentially experimenting from the lab to the industrial scale and testing a wide range of conditions increases our confidence to extrapolate. Early in our development program, we want to know if we can repeat results. In later development stages, we deliberately differentiate and vary the conditions to better define the operational space. We continue learning from observational studies[1] during commercial manufacture of the developed product.

Looking back over months or years, one can see the broader picture of developing the product from laboratory to scale-up

1 We conduct experimental studies during the product development stages to determine which factors influence the response. We deliberately change the factors and evaluate what happens to specific responses. We choose some factors to study, hold others constant, and ignore others. Experimentation implies the analyst's active participation in the data collection through deliberate changes in the factor settings.

We conduct observational studies to collect data on the responses during routine manufacturing. We assume the manufacturing will be consistent and predictable by holding the factors within a range. When the manufacturing is not consistent, we experiment with identifying the issues and improving. Observational studies imply the analyst's somewhat passive involvement in the data collection without deliberate changes in the factor settings.

to commercial supplies. The process is like a stained-glass window: You step back to gain the full effect.

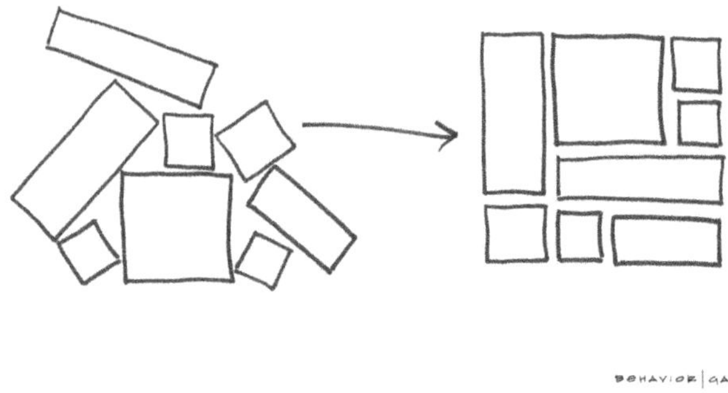

NOTES

The constant interplay between idea and experimentation is an ongoing back-and-forth motion between the drafting, correction, and generation of the concept until we arrive at models that meet our needs. The point of organizing experiments is not to ensure a unique product development pathway but to converge to a correct solution. Many scientists have expressed these ideas, such as Bernard C. (1957). *An Introduction to the Study of Experimental Medicine.* NY: Dover, and Medawar, P.B. (1982). *Pluto's Republic.* 99–103, 129–135. Oxford: Oxford University Press.

The most eloquent exposition was by Box, G.E.P. (1999). Statistics as a Catalyst to Learning by Scientific Method Part II — A discussion. *Journal of Quality Technology* 31: 16–29; (2001). Statistics for Discovery. *Journal of Applied Statistics* 28: 285–299, and (co-authored with Draper, N.R. 1987). *Empirical Model-Building and Response Surfaces.* New York: Wiley. (with Kulahci, M. 2003). Catalysis of discovery and development in engineering and industry. *Quality Engineering* 15 (3): 513–517.

Ehrenberg, A.S.C. (1975) has written widely on deliberately varying the conditions during replication in *Data Reduction*. NY: Wiley. (with Lindsay, R.M. 1993). The design of replicated studies. *The American Statistician* 47: 217–228.

Ehrenberg, A.S.C. (1990). A Hope for the Future of Statistics: MSoD. *The American Statistician* 44: 47–68.

Fisher, R.A. (1952). Sequential experimentation. *Biometrics* 8 (3): 183–187.

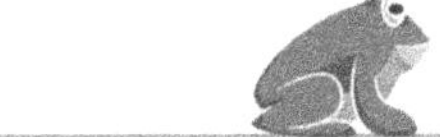

3

What Are the Stages of Drug Product Development?

Pharmaceutical programs include preclinical, clinical, drug substance, drug product, analytical testing, and manufacturing, among other critical activities.

The chemistry manufacturing and control (CMC) sections in a pharmaceutical product application to health agencies include drug substance, product, analytical testing, and manufacturing activities. CMC starts during the drug candidate selection phase and continues through post-approval and beyond. The CMC data package shows the link between the drug product used in the clinical studies and the commercial drug product available to patients. The CMC data package is not prescriptive but tailored to the drug substance, product, and analytical methods. Figure 3.1 shows the CMC development activities from the preclinical stage until filing a new drug application. We will summarize the drug product development activities in this chapter.

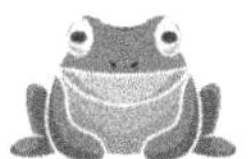

Function or Activity	Preclinical	Phase 1 Clinical Trials	Phase 2 Clinical Trials	Phase 3 Clinical Trials	Filings
Regulatory CMC	Pre - IND meeting	IND/IMPD for Phase 1 Update IND/IMPD for Phase 2	Decision : Fast track, Breakthrough or Accelerated submission IND/IMPD for Phase 3 Discussions on DS starting materials End of phase 2 meeting Additional meeting requests by sponsor	Pre-NDA Meeting DS filing documents DP filing documents Analytical filing documents Lock DS starting materials	CMC filing within NDA Pre-approval inspections
Chemistry Manufacturing and Controls (CMC)					
Chemistry and Process Development Drug Substance Manufacturing	Synthesis GLP Tox batch Salt Selection IND route Polymorph selection	GMP Batch GMP resupply Process development	Toxicology support DS process defined Agree on sourcing strategy Registration stability batches Track and define impurities	Toxicology support Validation protocol Validation batches	
Drug Product Development Drug Product Manufacturing	Support Toxicology Support DS Clinical formulation development	Clinical trial material Clinical trial material resupply	Process characterization Define commercial product Process scale-up	Registration stability batches Process robustness Commercial scale-up Validation protocol	Validation batches
Analytical Development	Method development Phase relevant validation Support DS and DP Stability studies	DS specification for Phase 1 DP specification for Phase 1 Stability studies for DS and DP	Method Refinement, Robustness, and Validation DS and DP specifications for Phase 3 Stability studies for DS and DP	Method transfer and Method validation Commercial DS and DP specifications Stability studies for DS and DP	

IND : investigational new drug; IMPD : investigational medicinal product dossier; NDA : new drug application; GLP : good laboratory practice; DS : drug susbtance; DP : drug product; Tox : toxicology; GMP : good manufacturing practice

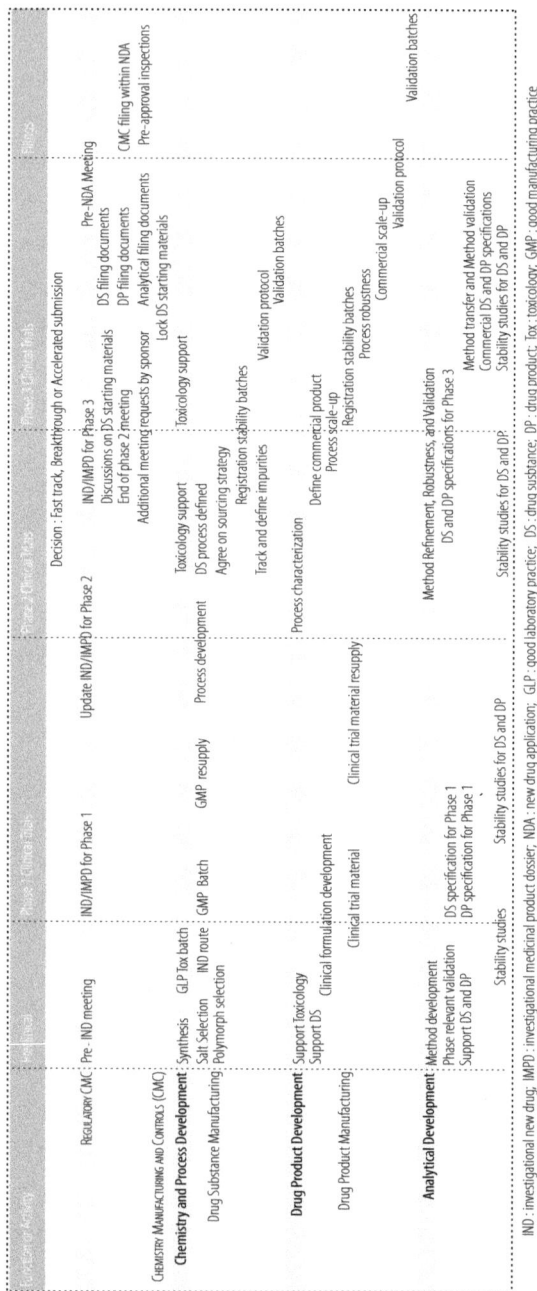

Figure 3.1: A simplified outline of how chemistry manufacturing and controls developmental activities fit in a pharmaceutical development program.

The stages of drug product development from the laboratory to pilot scale to industrial production drug products include

Drug product profile

Product development

Process development

- Early process development
- Process characterization studies
- Process robustness studies

Registration stability batches

Scale-up and transfer to commercial site

Validation batches

We briefly summarize the product profile, product, and process development stages.

Drug product profile

A drug product profile describes the dosage form design and performance needs. We evaluate, define, and revise the drug product qualities during the development and registration stages. The product's essential qualities influence performance, quality, safety, and efficacy. Tables 3.1 and 3.2 show the product profile and product details for a modified release oral dosage form.

Table 3.1: Drug product profile for a modified release oral dosage form

Characteristic	Description	Upside profile
Therapeutic area	Immunology	Immunology
Population	Adult	Pediatric
Administration	Oral	Oral
Frequency	Twice a day	Once a day
Handling	Cannot subdivide	Not applicable

Table 3.2: Drug product details for a modified release dosage form

Characteristic	Description	Qualities	Influences
Dosage form	Modified release tablet	Dissolution	Safety and efficacy
Strengths	25 mg, 50 mg	Assay Content uniformity	Safety and efficacy
Clinical image	Coated caplets with no scoring	Tablet appearance	Patient compliance
Commercial image	Coated caplets with no scoring	Tablet appearance	Patient compliance
Storage	Room temperature	Assay Related substances Dissolution	Safety and efficacy

Product development

Drug product design depends on drug substance chemistry, forms, solubility, solid state, solution stability, chemical stability, handling, and administration routes. Characterizing the drug substance's physical and chemical properties and developing the early product occurs in the laboratory. Early formulation studies include compatibility experiments that probe the chemical stability between the excipient, drug substance, and components. Experimenters store the samples at accelerated conditions for a short period and monitor the assay and impurities. At early stages, milligrams or a few grams of drug substance are available for clinical product development. The experimenter chooses an experimental design to fit the constraint.

Additional experiments define the type components and percentage of excipients. The in vitro quality measures (Table 3.1) and stability studies identify the clinical and commercial products. The experimenter decides the physical and chemical characterization studies helpful in developing the drug product.

Process development

Phase 2 and, on occasion, Phase 3 clinical supplies come from early scale-up studies. Pilot-scale and laboratory studies develop the know-how to make the product and supply Phase 3 and registration stability studies. These studies help design commercial production and gather information for the registration dossier. Industrial scale-up activities supply site registration stability studies. This scale-up helps design the qualification batches, followed by routine commercial supplies and distribution.

Early process development

The objective is to identify a process and the initial operating ranges. We make the prototype(s) using one or two production methods at target conditions. Experience helps choose the target conditions. Responses include the in vitro quality measures (Table 3.2) and stability. This work enables the manufacturing of clinical supplies, the initial building of process knowledge, and the analysis of clinical supply batches for trends.

Process characterization studies

The objective is to outline a risk assessment table, characterize the process, and complete initial scale-up trials. Process characterization studies at laboratory and pilot scales gather data to determine which factors influence the quality measures. The studies include equipment and formulation parameters (temperature, pressure, pH, drug substance particle size, and excipient grade) on quality measures. Package selection studies identify the material and arrangement for the product. Early experiments on dissolution method discrimination at this stage help define the dissolution method for registration studies.

Process robustness studies

Reviewing the earlier process studies' data helps decide the studies for commercial scale-up. We include scale-dependent factors to support the transfer to commercial equipment and sites. The robustness studies confirm the working or proven acceptable ranges and identify the process controls to produce the product. Experimenters evaluate drug substances and excipients of varying physical qualities and packaging studies if necessary. The study results will help update the initial risk assessment.

Registration stability batches

To determine the product shelf life, we conduct long-term stability studies of the product in the container closure system for the marketed product. Three primary batches are usually manufactured at pilot scale using different batches of drug substances when possible and representing the commercial manufacturing process. The quality and specification should define the product intended for marketing. Stability studies are performed on each strength and container size of the drug product unless bracketing is applied.

Commercial scale-up

The scale-up at the industrial site confirms the equipment settings. Experiments define the target settings; acceptable operating range of factors like pressure, temperature, and stirring speed; and the procedure for controlling the equipment settings and demonstrating the factors' importance. If necessary, the commercial site will produce site-specific stability batches. We complete the risk assessment before the validation batches.

Validation batches

Validation batches are commercial-scale batches manufactured consecutively to determine if the process is adequate for reproducible commercial manufacturing.

Programs seldom follow a straightforward path in the stages of drug product development. Nevertheless, technical or business-related issues are ever present.

- Issues about drug substance, product performance, analytical methods, quality, and production are always present.
- We may have to develop a clinical-stage drug with an unsatisfactory formula or an unacceptable process needing constant surveillance.
- We have a sped-up clinical development and approval timeline, leaving inadequate time to complete all the development and registration studies.

Table 3.3: Drug product development stages, and the proposed manufacturing scales

	Product/ Formulation development	Early process development	Process characterization studies	Initial scale-up	Process robustness studies	Transfer to commercial site and scale-up	Validation batches
Objective	Develop the product/ formulation.	Identify a process for clinical supplies.	Evaluate the effect of process and formulation parameters on the quality measures.	Scale-up	Evaluate process robustness with formulation parameters on quality measures.	Industrial scale-up and support the parameter ranges for commercial manufacture.	Confirm the process parameters for commercial manufacturing.
Scale	Laboratory	Laboratory	Laboratory and pilot plant	Pilot plant	Laboratory and pilot plant	Industrial site	Industrial site

Table 3.3 summarizes the drug product development stages.

Our flexibility and freedom to significantly change or radically adapt decreases as the project progresses from the early clinical stages to commercial stages (Figure 3.2). The reasons are time, money, regulatory constraints, pivotal trials using the product, and commitments at the commercial facility.

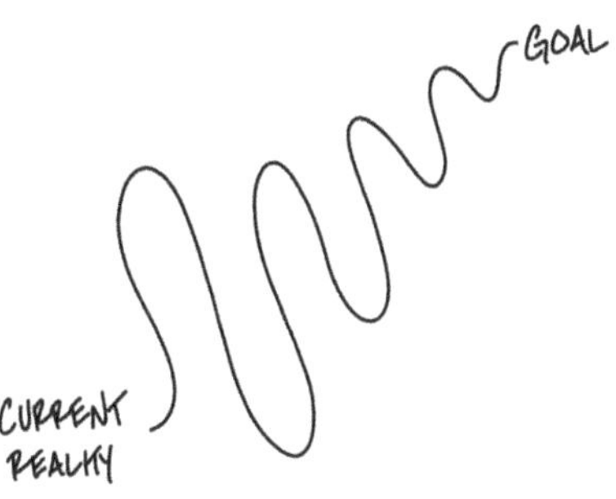

Figure 3.2: Our options and ability to change decrease from product development to commercial manufacture.

Understanding drug substance and product properties, material qualities, analytical methods, production, packaging, regulations, and equipment help resolve technical issues. Once we build an accurate mental map of the system we are trying to navigate, we can identify the blank spots. Knowing the end goal of a qualified commercial output helps us identify the gaps in product development data, technical trials, and analysis that need addressing for the commercial product and writing the new drug application filing. Sequential design thinking, subject matter, and risk assessment help us think about what to do.

Comparing data between the development stages enables us to develop a valuable history for setting working ranges, production specifications, identifying controls, managing risks, and registration filing.

NOTES

Campbell, J.J. (2018). *Understanding Pharma: The Professional's Guide to How Pharmaceutical and Biotech Companies Really Work.* NC: Syneos Health.

The U.S. Drug Administration Center for Drug Evaluation and Research (CDER) issued the "Guidance for Industry Process Validation: General Principles and Practices" in 2011. This guidance outlines the general principles and approaches that the Federal Drug Administration considers appropriate elements of process validation for drug manufacture or products. Process validation takes place over the life cycle of the product and has three stages:

Stage 1: Process design: We define the commercial manufacturing process based on knowledge gained through development and scale-up activities.

Stage 2: Process qualification: We evaluate the process design to determine if the process will support reproducible commercial manufacturing.

Stage 3: Continued process verification: We gain assurance that the process remains in a state of control during routine production.

https://www.fda.gov/files/drugs/published/Process-Validation--General-Principles-and-Practices.pdf

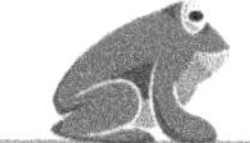

4

COMPARED WITH WHAT?

Experimenters compare different sets of readings when analyzing and interpreting. They compare trials with and without treatment and new data with existing data to determine if it is lower, higher, or the same. The discovery of the first noble gas, argon, by John Strutt (Rayleigh) and William Ramsay in 1895 is an illustrative example; it was awarded the Nobel Prize in 1904.

The process began when Rayleigh found small differences in the density of nitrogen purified by different methods. Those other methods led to varying quantities of nitrogen and different proportions of nitrogen, and an unexpected atmospheric gas. In a later investigation, he examined the mass of nitrogen from various sources (Table 4.1).

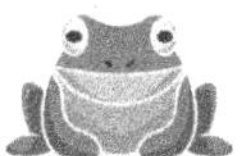

We order Rayleigh's original data in descending order (Table 4.1). To do so, we first analyze any time dependency between the experimental data (Figure 4.1). Placing data to be compared in columns helps us see patterns and exceptions. Table 4.1 includes residuals, the individual values minus the average of all the data.

Table 4.1: Weight in grams of nitrogen from the air and other sources including nitric oxide (NO), nitrous oxide (N_2O), ammonium nitrate (NH_4NO_3), ammonium nitrite (NH_4NO_2)

Order of data collection	Date	Source	Weight	Residuals[1] (weight-average)
15	Feb 01, 1894	Air	2.31028	0.00584
13	Jan 27, 1894	Air	2.31024	0.00580
5	Dec 12, 1893	Air	2.31017	0.00573
14	Jan 30, 1894	Air	2.31010	0.00566
7	Dec 19, 1893	Air	2.31010	0.00566
8	Dec 22, 1893	Air	2.31001	0.00557
6	Dec 14, 1893	Air	2.30986	0.00542
4	Dec 06, 1893	NO	2.30182	−0.00262
1	Nov 29, 1893	NO	2.30143	−0.00301
10	Dec 28, 1893	N_2O	2.29940	−0.00504
2	Dec 02, 1893	NO	2.29890	−0.00554
12	Jan 13, 1894	NH_4NO_3	2.29889	−0.00555
9	Dec 26, 1893	N_2O	2.29869	−0.00575
11	Jan 09, 1894	NH_4NO_2	2.29849	−0.00595
3	Dec 05, 1893	NO	2.29816	−0.00628
		Average	**2.30444**	

[1] Models are an attempt to mimic reality, and residuals are discrepancies between reality and the model. Here the average is the model, and the residual is the difference between the individual weights and the average.

Examining the results of Rayleigh's measurements from various sources reveals a clear difference between the two sets of data (Table 4.1, Figure 4.2). The difference is more significant than

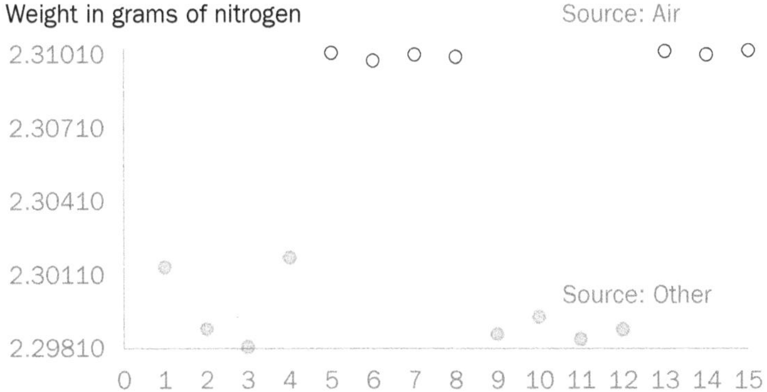

Figure 4.1: Plotting the order of Rayleigh's measurements does not show any time dependency.

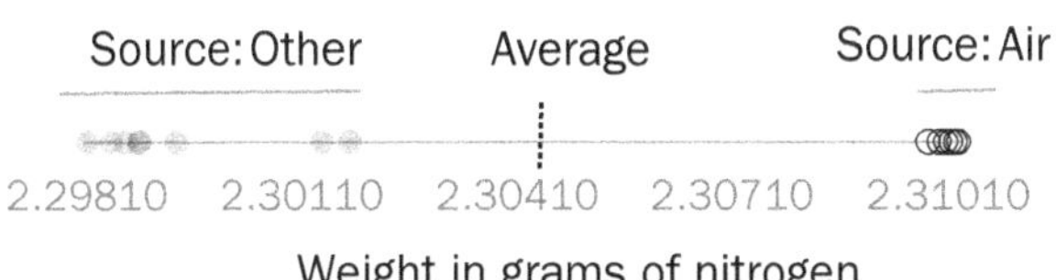

Figure 4.2: The dot plot of the nitrogen weights shows the differences between the two sources.

the experimental measurement error. Rayleigh and Ramsay isolated the then-unknown gas, compared the spectrum to existing substances, and examined the periodic table placement. Based on existing knowledge, Ramsay identified that it belonged to a new family of inert gases. By the end of the century, Ramsay had isolated helium and discovered neon, krypton, and xenon.

Most experiments follow the same logic of making comparisons as the discovery of argon. Learning through comparisons is human.

We know how to make comparisons from our pre-school days when we decide if shapes are the same or different: O O □ O; in our adult lives when we compare our home and work lives, the office and the factory floor.

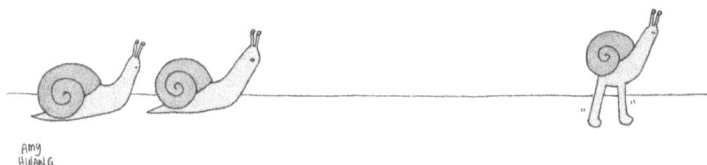

"I'd be fast, too, if I had legs that long."

Rayleigh's experiment had two factors, the source with two levels—air, and the other, which includes nitric oxide (NO), nitrous oxide (N_2O), ammonium nitrate (NH_4NO_3), ammonium nitrite (NH_4NO_2), and the reducing agent with two levels—iron and copper. We can compare multiple factors with two or more levels simultaneously through factorial experiments. The next chapter introduces factorial experiments and shows how experimental design acts as a same-or-different machine.

NOTES

Lord Rayleigh, (1894). On an anomaly encountered in determinations of the density of nitrogen gas. *Proceedings of the Royal Society of London* 55: 340–344.

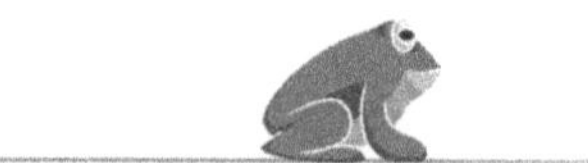

5

What Can We Learn From Four Experiments?

Experimenters want to find out the effect of factors at certain levels on a response of interest. Which factors at what levels and which responses to measure come from subject matter.

- Factors are variables whose effect we study. They can be quantitative or qualitative. Quantitative factors include pH, temperature, number of blender rotations, capsule fill rate, capsule pin settings, roll force, roll gap, tablet press speed, compression force, spray rates, and atomization pressure. Qualitative factors include excipient type, excipient grade, drug substance forms, and polymer type. Think of them as the usual suspects.
- The experimenter chooses the desired levels, or values, for each of the factors they wish to study. For example, they might assign two pHs (pH 4.5 and pH 6.8) and two temperatures (50°C and 70°C) for quantitative factors;

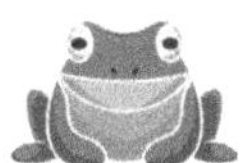

two types of fillers (cellulose and lactose) and two types of polymers (hydroxypropyl cellulose and methylcellulose) for qualitative factors.

- Responses are a measure of product and process performance. These might include assay, impurity, degradant, percentage moisture, percentage dissolved in dissolution testing, dosage form weight, and percentage weight gain of coated tablets.

Factorial designs run all combinations of the levels to examine the effects of the factors and potential interactions. The simple two-level factorial designs are practical because geometric displays, elementary arithmetic, and graphical analysis help analyze the data. They are the building blocks of sequential experimentation (Figure 1.1). The following example shows how Yesim at Hill Therapeutics used two-level experimental designs within a sequential framework to develop a modified release product.

Developing a modified release product

Yesim, from the drug product department, had to develop a modified release product for an insoluble crystalline drug. The company was running a Phase 2 clinical study for a twice-a-day immediate release dosage form. There were discussions of developing a once-a-day product to increase competitive advantage and possible patient compliance. After much debate on commercial strategy, patient compliance, and clinical and regulatory risk, the management asked the project team to develop a once-a-day drug product bioequivalent to the twice-a-day product in the clinical studies. The once-a-day product would be a modified release product, and the technical team had to decide on the initial in vitro criteria.

After discussions based on existing data, opinion, simulation, and experience, Yesim, Mae from the analytical development department, and Xia from the clinical pharmacology department estimated the initial criteria for the in vitro dissolution of the modified release product (Table 5.1). The team planned to conduct an exploratory pharmacokinetic study in healthy volunteers after Yesim's team identified the prototypes meeting the in vitro dissolution and stability criteria.

Yesim identified two polymers (factors) with two grades (levels) for each polymer, given the drug's physical and chemical characteristics and the target dissolution profile. Table 5.1 outlines the background.

Table 5.1: Outlining the objective, experimental factors, levels, and responses for developing a modified release product

Objective	Identify the polymer combination to meet the needed in vitro dissolution profile.		
Drug substance	A water-insoluble crystalline drug.		
Strength(s)	90 mg		
Factors	**Level (–)**	**Level (+)**	**Information**
Polymer 1	Low molecular weight	High molecular weight	Polymers are in the FDA inactive ingredient database.
Polymer 2	Low viscosity	Medium viscosity	Polymer 1: Polymer 2 will be 50:50
Response Variable	**Measurement**	**Information**	**Initial criteria**
Percentage drug release over time.	Dissolution	USP type 2 apparatus, 75 rpm, 1,000 mL phosphate buffer pH6.8, 37.0 ± 0.5°C	≤15% at 2 hours 40% at 4 hours 75% at 8 hours
Stability	Related substances	Reverse phase HPLC	% individual <0.2 % total <0.6%

USP: United States Pharmacopeia; HPLC: High-performance liquid chromatography.

Yesim, with the help of Rao, the statistician, designed a two-level, two-factor, or 2^2 factorial design (two polymer types x two molecular weights). Table 5.2 displays the design.

Table 5.2: A 2^2 factorial design to evaluate the effect of polymer type and polymer grade on the dissolution profile for a modified release product

Trials	Order	Polymer 1	Polymer 2	Geometric representation Numbers at vertices are trials
1	3	–	–	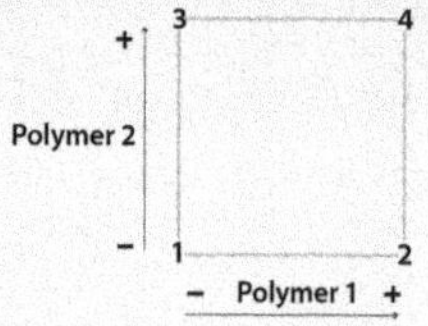
2	2	+	–	
3	4	–	+	
4	1	+	+	
	–	Low molecular weight	Low viscosity	
	+	High molecular weight	Medium viscosity	

- A trial is an experiment with factor and level combinations.
- Randomization lessens the systematic effect of uncontrolled or unknown factors that could change over time. Examples are ambient temperature, humidity, operators, equipment wear and tear, and lot-to-lot difference.
- The Order column is the order in which the experimenter completes the trials. Randomization decides the order.

The factorial design is an excellent same-or-different machine. The square represents Polymers 1 and 2 in a 2^2 design (Table 5.2). The corners of the square represent the experimental conditions. Yesim makes four comparisons, corresponding to the square's four borders for the response, and considers:

- On average, are results the same or different on the left-hand side as on the right-hand side (the main effect of Polymer 1's molecular weight)?
- On average, are results the same or different on the top as on the bottom (the main effect of Polymer 2's viscosity)?

- Comparing the square's diagonals shows the possibility of interaction between the factors. An interaction comparison will reveal whether the differences produced by Polymer 1 are the same or different when Polymer 2 is changed.

Coding the levels of a factor using the minus and plus signs

We use the minus sign to represent the factor's low level and a plus sign for its high level. Using minus and plus signs to describe the levels of the factor is a way of coding the levels. Representing the levels in coded units has several advantages. By coding, we scale all the effects the same way and enable comparison. Further, using this coding, the columns shown in Table 5.2 are orthogonal (see notes at the end of the chapter), and effects can be estimated independently of each other. Two-level factorial designs are orthogonal. The minus and plus coding also simplify the effect calculations. Effect refers to the influence of the factor(s) on the response.

For a qualitative factor, the minus and plus signs represent the experimenter's descriptive levels. For a quantitative factor, the minus and plus signs are the factor's low and high values. As an example, consider drying temperature as a factor. Figure 5.1 visually shows how we go from original to coded units for various temperatures. For example, 50°C, which is the low temperature value, is -1; 70°C, which is the high temperature

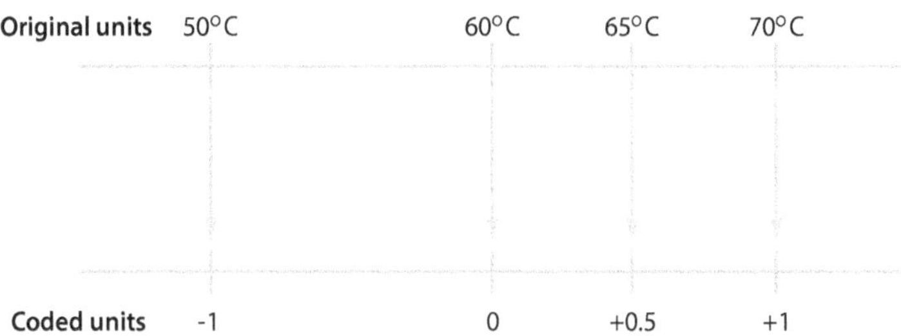

Figure 5.1: A visual relating original temperature units in degrees Celsius to the coded units from -1 to +1.

value, is +1; 60°C, which is halfway between 50°C and 70°C, is 0; and 65°C, which is halfway between 60°C and 70°C, is +0.5.

We calculate the coded values for other temperature values using

$$T_{coded} = \frac{T_{celcius} - \left[\frac{70 + 50}{2}\right]}{\frac{70 - 50}{2}} \qquad (5.1)$$

For example, for 50°C the coded unit is $\frac{50 - 60}{10} = -1$

Experimental data from the first set of experiments

Table 5.3 shows the dissolution data from the first set of experiments.

Table 5.3: The average dissolution profile data (n = 6 dosage units) from experiments evaluating the effect of polymer type and polymer grade in developing a modified release product

				Percentage dissolved over time, hours						
Trials	Order	Polymer 1	Polymer 2	1	2	4	6	8	10	12
1	3	–	–	32	60	91	98	98	99	99
2	2	+	–	32	55	80	98	99	99	99
3	4	–	+	23	41	60	71	85	96	98
4	1	+	+	23	38	51	63	75	85	95
			Criteria		≤15	30 to 50		65 to 80		

No issues arose in other measured responses on the dosage form, including weight uniformity, content uniformity, assay, related substances, and water content. Yesim packaged 30 tablets of each prototype in 30 cc high-density polyethylene bottles with an induction seal. Her colleague in the stability department placed the packaged and labeled bottles in stability chambers maintained at 25°C/60%RH and 40°C/75%RH for a 6-month stability study.

Analysis

In most experiments, the response is a single number for each experiment. The data in Table 5.3, however, shows a response measured over time. Figure 5.2 shows the dissolution profile or percentage dissolved over time.

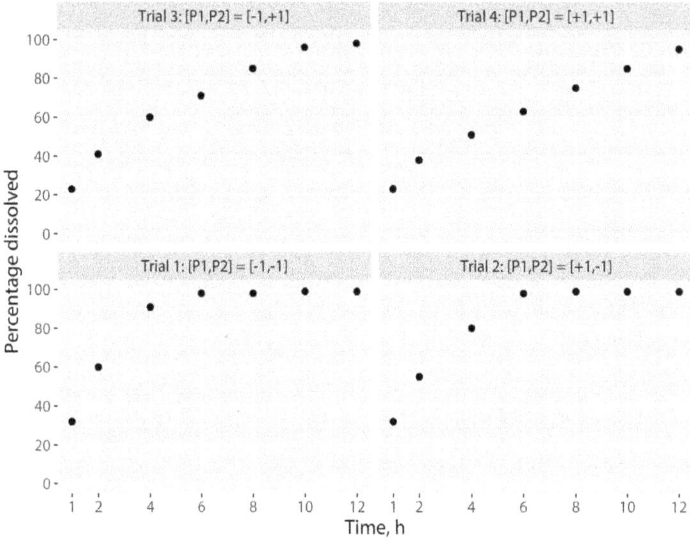

Figure 5.2: Dissolution profile from four experiments evaluating the effect of polymer type and polymer grade in developing a modified release product. The data points represent the average (n = 6 dosage units) percentage dissolved at individual time points. Polymer 2 in this experimental design extends the duration of drug release and reduces the release rate from the tablets (Trials 3 and 4).

The typical diffusion and erosion of tablets result in similar profile shapes. But what's the response? We can focus on a single time point and study the polymers' influence on the percentage of dissolution at a specific time and analyze each time point. However, the rate that will dictate the percentage of drug dissolved over time for a modified release dissolution profile is actually of interest. The first step of the analysis is finding and fitting a relevant dissolution versus. time model to the profiles. We use the model's parameters, including slope, which vary from experiment to experiment as the new responses. In this case, we propose the following model for the percentage dissolved over time:

$$\%\ dissolved = a_0 - a_1 e^{-a_2 \times (time - t_0)} \qquad (5.2)$$

where a_0, a_1, and a_2 are the parameters to estimate and define the profile characteristics we see in Figure 5.3. t_0 in hours is the potential delay in the dissolution. For the design in Table 5.3, we assume t_0 is zero.

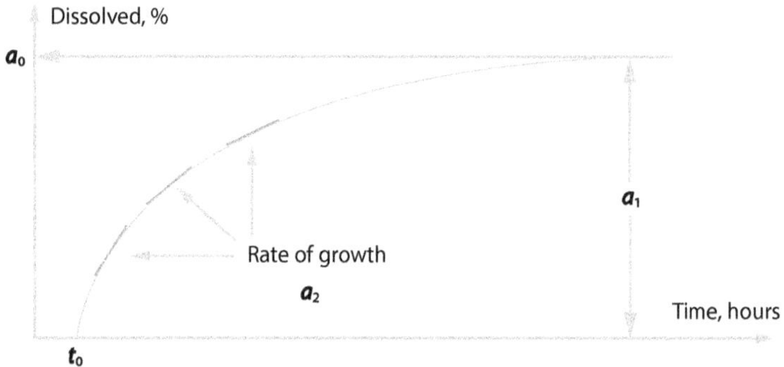

Figure 5.3: A schematic representation of a dissolution profile showing the parameters from the model % *dissolved* $= a_0 - a_1 e^{-a_2 \times (time - t_0)}$ (exponential growth with a negative rate of growth a_2).

In the model, a_0 indicates the asymptotic value that percentage dissolved will eventually take, a_0 - a_1 represents the percentage dissolved at time zero, and a_2 is the rate with which the dissolution occurs. We can simplify the model shown in (5.2) by setting a_0 to 100, assuming 100% asymptotic dissolution, and a_1 to 100, suggesting that dissolution should be precisely zero percent at time zero. Therefore, we can reduce the modeling to estimate a_2 for each profile and use that as the experiments' response. We summarize any profile with this single number and study the effects of polymer type and grade on dissolution rate. Please note that we could estimate all parameters and use all of them as responses. However, reducing the entire profile into a single number makes sense and simplifies the analysis in this specific case. Our objective for the model is not to provide a detailed picture of reality but rather to capture the key factors that give insight.

We can estimate a_2 by fitting a nonlinear regression model of the form:

$$\frac{\%\ dissolved - a_0}{-a_1} = \left(\frac{\%\ dissolved - 100}{-100}\right) = e^{-a_2 \times time} + \varepsilon$$

where ε represents the experimental error. The experimental error may be due to unknown factors in the manufacture of the tablets and measurement uncertainties. We do not focus our attention on the experimental error at this early stage. The reader will recall e refers to the base of the natural logarithm, also known as Euler's number. We linearize the profile by taking the natural $\log\left(\frac{\%\ dissolved - 100}{-100}\right)$ or $\ln\left(\frac{100 - \%\ dissolved}{100}\right)$.

As a result, the slope of the regression line going through the (0,0) coordinates will represent $-a_2$, the calculated dissolution rate. Figure 5.4 is an illustration of this linearization.

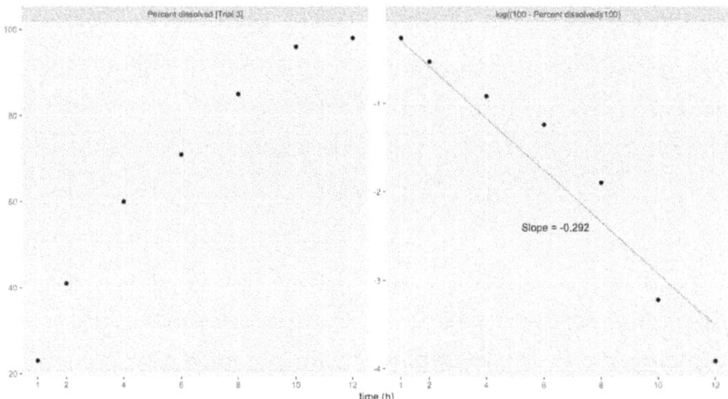

Figure 5.4: The left panel shows the dissolution profile for tablets from Trial 3 (Table 5.3). The data points represent the percentage dissolved at individual time points. The right panel shows the data after linearization. The slope from the linearization represents the rate constant a_2.

Table 5.4 shows the estimated a_2 values using the nonlinear model. Next, we use a_2 in (5.2) to calculate the predicted percentage dissolved over time for each trial and display this as a dotted line in Figure 5.5.

Table 5.4: The estimated rate of dissolution a_2 for experiments evaluating the effect of polymer type and polymer grade on the dissolution profile (For the statistical analysis of the estimation of these rates, please see the book's website. datatodecision.org)

Trials	Order	Polymer 1	Polymer 2	$-a_2$
1	3	–	–	0.476
2	2	+	–	0.418
3	4	–	+	0.241
4	1	+	+	0.190

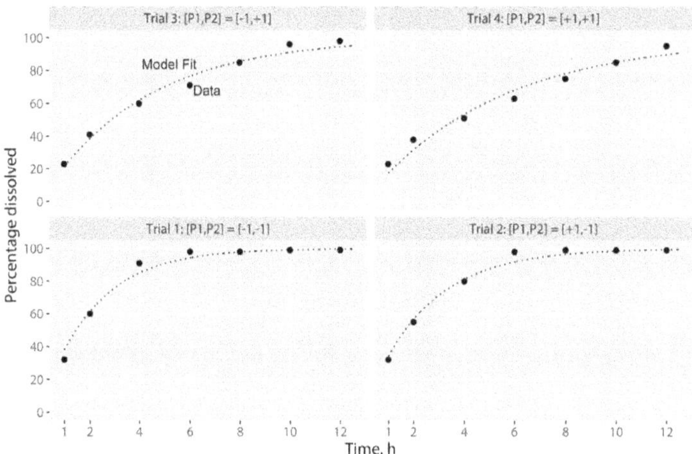

Figure 5.5: Dissolution profile from four experiments evaluating the effect of polymer type and polymer grade in developing a modified release product. The data points represent the percentage dissolved at individual time points. The dotted line is the model fit to % *dissolved* = $a_0 - a_1 e^{-a_2 \times (time - t_0)}$. $a_0 = 100$, $a_1 = 100$, $t_0 = 0$.

In these experiments, the main effects and interaction effects are of interest.

- The main effects represent the influence of each of the polymers individually. The difference of the average response at the high and low levels for each polymer estimates the main effect.
- An interaction effect means the effect of a factor on the response will depend on the level of the other factor. We discuss the effect of a factor for a given level of the other factor and avoid interpreting the effect of each factor separately. For example, interaction between the polymers measures the change in Polymer 1 effect as we vary Polymer 2 or the change in Polymer 2 effect as we vary levels of Polymer 1.

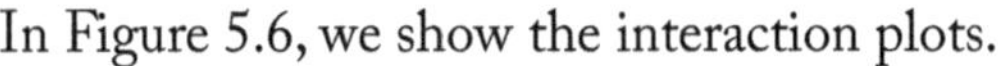
In Figure 5.6, we show the interaction plots.

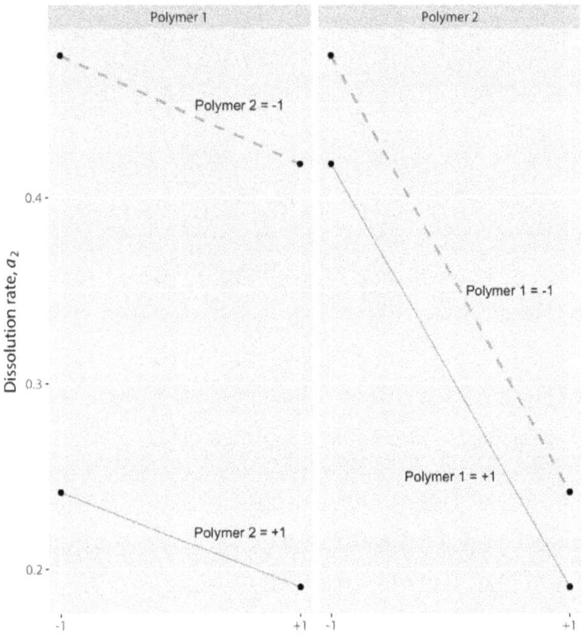

Figure 5.6: Interaction plots of dissolution rate a_2. The dotted lines represent the low level of either Polymer 1 or 2, and the solid lines represent the high level of either Polymer 1 or 2. There is no interaction between the polymers.

Table 5.3 represents an un-replicated 2^2 design. We do not have enough data to establish the statistical significance of the effects. A statistically significant result does not mean an absolute significance and comes with a level of confidence, such as 95%, in that claim, and (100%—the confidence level) refers to the probability of potentially being wrong when declaring statistical significance. A practically meaningful result affects how, when, or where we use the product even without statistical significance (see notes at the end of the chapter). We limit our analysis to a visual assessment of the interaction plots in Figure 5.6. The parallel lines in the interaction plots suggest no interactions between the polymers. Two factors interact if the effect of one factor is different at different levels of another factor. A strong interaction effect would result in lines with different slopes in magnitude or sign or both in an interaction plot. We can perform a relative assessment of the main effects by studying the slopes of the lines in Figure 5.6. We tentatively infer that Polymer 2 has a greater effect on the dissolution rate than Polymer 1 as the slopes in the plot for Polymer 2 are steeper than the slopes for Polymer 1. This is tentative, as it is not concluded through statistical analysis.

Interpretation

- We include Polymer 2 in future experiments because it influences the rate and extent of the dissolution profile.
- Combining the high molecular weight of Polymer 1 and medium viscosity of Polymer 2 produces a release profile closer to the criteria (Trial 4, Order 1 in Table 5.3).
- However, no combination met the 2-hour release criterion of ≤15%. Yesim suggested using a pH-dependent coating to meet this criterion.
- Therefore, Yesim conjectured using only Polymer 2 and a pH-dependent coating could result in a release profile longer than 12 hours. Hence, they decided to include less than 20% of Polymer 1 low molecular weight or Polymer 2 low viscosity grade to weaken the tablet matrix and allow for a 12-hour dissolution profile. Yesim discussed this with Cliff from the technical operations department, and they agreed to use Polymer 2 low viscosity grade based on the ease of sourcing from one supplier. The supplier also had two plants in different geographical locations, reducing the supply chain risk.

What to do next

Design follow-up experiments to reduce the percentage of drug released at 2 hours to ≤15%:

- Evaluate different percentages [7 and 17] of a pH-dependent polymer coating.
- Evaluate different proportions [8:92 and 16:74] of Polymer 2: low viscosity (P2LV) and medium viscosity (P2MV).
- Implement a two-stage dissolution method: exposing the tablets to 0.1N hydrochloric acid for 2 hours, followed by dissolution in a buffer media with sampling points until 10 hours have elapsed in the buffer media.

Experimental data from a second set of experiments

Table 5.5 shows the dissolution data from a second set of experiments.

Table 5.5: The average dissolution profile data (n = 6) from experiments evaluating the effect of polymer proportions (P2LV: P2MV) and percentage pH coating in developing a modified release product. The calculated dissolution rate constant a_2 is from % *dissolved* $= a_0 - a_1 e^{-a_2 \times (time - t_0)}$. $a_0 = 100, a_1 = 100, t_0 = 1$

				Percentage dissolved over time, hours							
Trials	Order	P2LV: P2MV	% pH coating	1	2	4	6	8	10	12	$-a_2$
1	4	−	−	0	15	60	84	93	97	98	0.315
2	2	+	−	0	17	56	78	87	93	96	0.278
3	1	−	+	0	3	25	46	66	80	95	0.150
4	3	+	+	0	12	40	65	80	90	96	0.211
	−	8:92	7								
	+	16:74	17								
			Criteria		≤15	30 to 50		65 to 80			

Analysis

We fit the model (5.2) and calculated the rate of dissolution a_2. We set t_0 to one hour in this case because the pH-sensitive polymer does not dissolve readily in 0.1N HCl but dissolves in the buffer media. Therefore, we are interested in the dissolution rate a_2 and the percent released at 2 hours in 0.1N HCl. We use 0.1N HCl because it simulates the environmental pH of the stomach. Two hours represents the stomach transit time.

From the fitted (dotted) lines in Figure 5.7, only trial three is close to meeting the target criteria from Table 5.3.

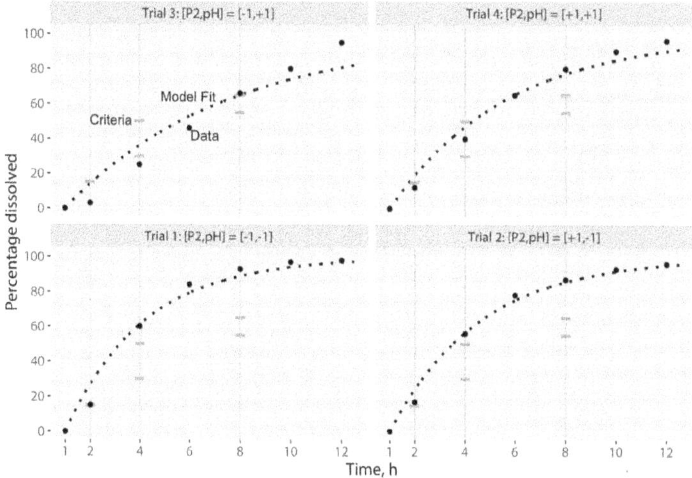

Figure 5.7: Dissolution profile from four experiments evaluating the effect of polymer proportions (P2LV: P2MV) and percentage of pH coating in developing a modified release product. The data points represent the percentage dissolved at individual time points. The dotted line is the model fit to % *dissolved* $= a_0 - a_1 e^{-a_2 \times (time - t_0)}$ • $a_0 = 100, a_1 = 100, t_0 = 1$.

Interpretation

Figures 5.8 and 5.9 show the interaction plots for a_2 and percentage dissolved at 2 hours from the experiments in Table 5.5.

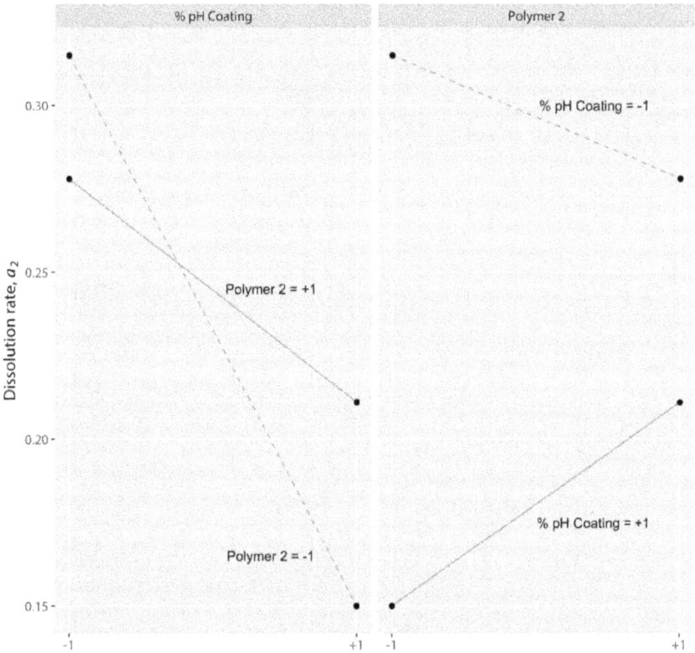

Figure 5.8: Interaction plots of dissolution rate a_2. The dotted lines represent the low level of either Polymer 2 or percentage of pH coating, and the solid lines represent the high level of either Polymer 2 or percentage of pH coating. There is a potential interaction between percentage of pH coating and Polymer 2.

The tentative conclusions we can draw are:

- The ratio of Polymer 2 and pH-sensitive coating interact so that the impact of Polymer 2 changes signs with the levels of pH-sensitive coating. The ratio of Polymer 2 can either increase or decrease the dissolution rate depending on the pH-sensitive coating.

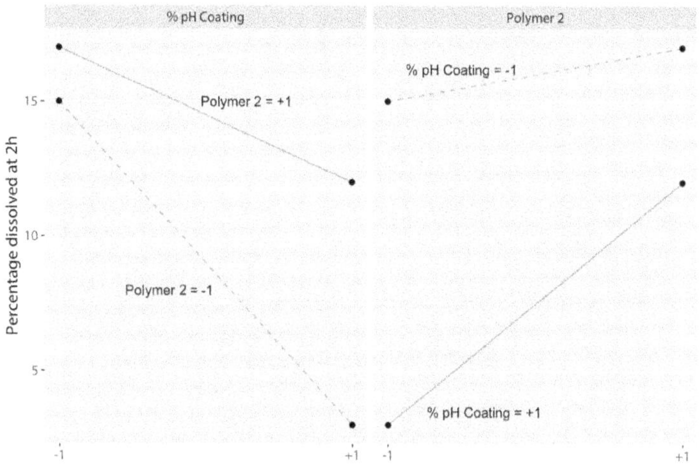

Figure 5.9: Interaction plots of percentage dissolved at Hour 2. The dotted lines represent the low level of either Polymer 2 or percentage of pH coating, and the solid lines represent the high level of either Polymer 2 or percentage of pH coating. There is a potential interaction between percentage of pH coating and Polymer 2.

- The potential interaction between the two factors makes it challenging to discuss the "main" effect of any factor, as the main effect of one factor changes with the levels of the other factor. Nonetheless, pH coating seems to lower the rate of dissolution. The pH-sensitive layer delays the start of drug release from the tablet, which negatively affects the rate. The magnitude of the delay depends on the ratio of Polymer 2. A higher amount of P2MV (P2LV: P2MV = 8:92) decreases the dissolution rate more when the pH-sensitive coating goes from 7% to 17%.
- As shown in Figure 5.9, the ratio of Polymer 2 and the percentage of pH-sensitive coating may also be interacting for the percentage released at 2 hours

since the lines are not parallel. This interaction effect means the effect of the polymer ratio on the percentage dissolved at 2 hours depends on the percentage of pH-sensitive coating. Put another way, the influence of the percentage of pH-sensitive coating depends on the ratio of Polymer 2. The ratio containing a higher percentage of medium viscosity Polymer (P2LM: P2MV = 8:92) with the coating containing a higher percentage (17%) of the pH-sensitive polymer gave a lower-than-expected percentage of drug dissolved at 2 hours.

What to do next

The next steps should include collecting dissolution data at 1, 2, 3, 4, 6, 8, 10, and 12 hours during dissolution testing for n = 12 tablets. The infinity point should be included after 12 hours to confirm a 100% release. This data collection will help the team set specifications for dissolution.

The project team discussed testing the product from Trials 3 and 4 (Table 5.5) in a pilot bioequivalence (BE) study with 12 healthy subjects. The pilot BE study would evaluate the prototypes, assess pharmacokinetic variability, determine the sample size to achieve adequate power for a future full-scale BE study, and choose sample collection times.

Pharmacokinetic study design to evaluate the modified release prototypes.

Bioavailability (BA) means the rate and extent to which the drug substance is absorbed from a drug product and becomes available in the living body. BA data provides information related to the pharmacokinetics of the drug. BE means there is no significant difference between two dosage forms in the rate and extent to which the drug substance becomes available at the drug action site when given under similar conditions in a designed study.

A BE study is designed to determine if the new drug product results in the same concentration in the blood as the reference product. Crossover designs are the designs of choice for BE trials. In a crossover design, each subject receives different treatments during different periods. That is, the subjects cross over from one treatment to another during the trial.

In our case, the project team decided to test three treatments in a pilot BE study—prototypes from Trials 3 and 4 (Table 5.5) and the twice-a-day clinical drug product, which serves as the reference product. Every subject in the pilot BE study receives all three products. The design (Table 5.6) was a three-period, three-treatment crossover design with 2 days washout period between the treatments.

Table 5.6: A pilot BE study design to evaluate the modified release prototypes with 12 subjects. A: Trial 3; B: Trial 4; C: twice-a-day clinical drug product

Sequence	Period 1	Period 2	Period 3
ABC	A	B	C
BCA	B	C	A
CAB	C	A	B

The clinical pharmacology team led by Xia completed the study. The results of the small pilot study would guide the team on future studies.

NOTES

A statistically significant effect does not mean that the observed difference is large or that the result is important. Thus, it may not be practically meaningful. Also, we cannot necessarily extrapolate results from the small scale to the large scale or from one site to another based on statistical significance. Instead, we rely on physical replication, which is the traditional route toward predictability. We show generalization and robustness when the results hold across equipment, differing batch sizes, sites, analytical methods, and operators.

In factorial experiments orthogonality ensures all the main effects and interactions can be independently estimated without entanglement.

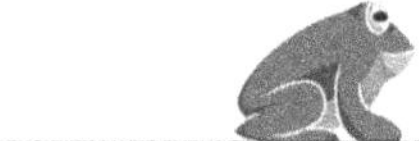

6

What Can We Learn From a Small Number of Experiments?

Two areas of investigation in the early stages are drug product development and manufacturing for human use. The tools used for the two areas differ since an experimenter is a detective during drug product development and a judge during drug product manufacturing for human use. The detective solves a problem sequentially using idea generation, informed observation, and directed experimentation. The exploratory approach to addressing the problem comes from considering the merest hints, slight differences among groups, and having a reasonable idea. Reasonable is not "right" since right and wrong are questions for confirmatory experiments rather than exploratory experiments.

During the exploratory and early stages of product development, small experimental designs and statistical data displays enable us to explore the experimental space and look at the data. Small

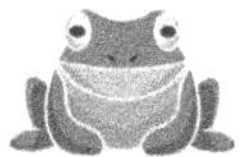

eight-run experimental designs are economical, easy to understand, and can evaluate multiple factors. Also, these designs build know-how sequentially, as sketched in Figure 1.1.

The two-level design with three factors, 2^3

The molecule candidate selection committee at Hill Therapeutics introduced a morpholine compound into the development pipeline. Yesim and Mae from the drug product development department and the analytical development department at Hill Therapeutics had to develop a Phase 1 clinical drug product for the morpholine compound.

Yesim and Mae met with Rao, the statistician, to design the development studies. After discussing the study with Yesim, Rao proposed eight experimental trials, or a 2^3 design. A geometric representation of the design shows each of the trials as the vertices of a cube. Table 6.1 shows this visually. Yesim would study the effect of three factors (process, lubricant, and diluent), represented by the letters P, L, and D, each at two levels, on drug product stability. Rao asked, what would be a practically meaningful difference between the trials? Yesim and Mae responded that a difference of 0.2% would be practically meaningful.

Table 6.1: The two-level design with three factors (2^3) to evaluate drug product stability of a morpholine compound

Trial	P	L	D	Cube plot with the trial numbers
1	–	–	–	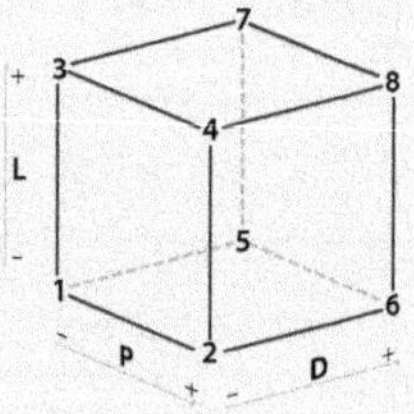
2	+	–	–	
3	–	+	–	
4	+	+	–	
5	–	–	+	
6	+	–	+	
7	–	+	+	
8	+	+	+	
–	Low	Low	Low	
+	High	High	High	

Rao explained that Yesim could calculate seven effects between the eight treatment combinations:

Three main effects, P, L, and D.

Three two-factor interactions, PL, PD, and LD.

One three-factor interaction, PLD.

Rao showed the seven effects by displaying the matrix for the effects in Table 6.2.

Table 6.2: The matrix of seven effects from a 2^3 design. Multiplying the signs of the factors gives the various interaction columns. For example, to get the PL (interaction) column, we multiply entry-wise the P and L columns

Trial	Factorial effect						
	P	L	D	PL	PD	LD	PLD
1	−	−	−	+	+	+	−
2	+	−	−	−	−	+	+
3	−	+	−	−	+	−	+
4	+	+	−	+	−	−	−
5	−	−	+	+	−	−	+
6	+	−	+	−	+	−	−
7	−	+	+	−	−	+	−
8	+	+	+	+	+	+	+

Experimental Data

Yesim carried out the experiments to evaluate the effect of excipients on the stability of the morpholine compound. The results shown in Table 6.3 are percentages of related substances after storing the product in loosened cap containers at 40°C/75%RH for 6 weeks.

Table 6.3: A 2^3 design to study the effect of the P, L, and D factors on the product stability of a morpholine compound stored at 40°C/75%RH for 6 weeks

Trial	Order	P	L	D	%RS
1	4	–	–	–	0.45
2	7	+	–	–	0.71
3	3	–	+	–	0.33
4	8	+	+	–	0.67
5	1	–	–	+	0.93
6	2	+	–	+	1.23
7	5	–	+	+	0.93
8	6	+	+	+	1.19
	–	DC	MS	M/S	
	+	WG	SA	M/L	

DC: direct compression; WG: wet granulation
MS: magnesium stearate; SA: stearic acid
M/S: microcrystalline cellulose/starch (70/30)
M/L: microcrystalline cellulose/anhydrous lactose (60/40)
%RS: percentage of related substances

Estimating the effects

In two-level factorial designs, we can calculate the effects as in one-factor-at-a-time experiments. Consider, for example, the main effect of P. We rearrange the eight experiments in Table 6.3 into four pairs of experiments where only the factor P changes levels within each pair, and the other factors remain at the same level. Hence these pairs can be separately used to estimate the effect of P, as shown in Table 6.4. But which of the four values should we use to estimate the effect? An intuitive option is to take the average of these four estimates, which is 0.29. Thus, one can calculate each effect by rearranging the runs in Table 6.3 as four pairs of one-factor-at-a-time experiments for that effect.

Table 6.4: Displaying the eight experiments from Table 6.3 as four pairs of one-factor-at-a-time experiments to estimate the effect of P

Trial	P	L	D	%RS	
1	–	–	–	0.45	Effect of P = 0.71 – 0.45 = 0.26
2	+	–	–	0.71	
3	–	+	–	0.33	Effect of P = 0.67 – 0.33 = 0.34
4	+	+	–	0.67	
5	–	–	+	0.93	Effect of P = 1.23 – 0.93 = 0.30
6	+	–	+	1.23	
7	–	+	+	0.93	Effect of P = 1.19 – 0.93 = 0.26
8	+	+	+	1.19	

In standard experimental design books, the effect of P is defined as the difference of the average response for the experiments for which P was at the high level and the average response for the experiments for which P was at the low level. Table 6.5 shows these averages for the design in Table 6.3 with the rearranged rows. The difference (0.95 – 0.66) is 0.29, which is the estimate we got earlier.

Table 6.5: Rearranging the experiments from Table 6.3 to show the conventional way to estimate the effect of P

Trial	P	L	D	%RS	
1	–	–	–	0.45	
3	–	+	–	0.33	Average $\%RS_{P=-1} = 0.66$
5	–	–	+	0.93	
7	–	+	+	0.93	
2	+	–	–	0.71	
4	+	+	–	0.67	Average $\%RS_{P=+1} = 0.95$
6	+	–	+	1.23	
8	+	+	+	1.19	

Mathematically the two approaches are equivalent:

$$\textit{Effect of P} = \frac{(0.71 - 0.45) + (0.67 - 0.33) + (1.23 - 0.093) + (1.19 - 0.93)}{4}$$

$$= \frac{(0.71 + 0.67 + 1.23 + 1.19)}{4} - \frac{(0.45 + 0.33 + 0.93 + 0.93)}{4}$$

$$= 0.95 - 0.66 = 0.29$$

The approach shown in Table 6.5 and commonly seen in books is not as intuitive as the one-factor-at-a-time experimentation approach shown in Table 6.4. Since we keep everything else constant and change only the level of the effect of interest, the change we observe in the response is due only to that effect. In the second approach, while we take the averages at each effect level, the other effects also change. So how can we assign those averages to that effect only? The answer lies in our (-1, +1) coding and the orthogonality of the two-level factorial design. Consider the rearranged design in Table 6.6, in which the first rows correspond to the low level of P and the last four to its high level. In taking the average of the first and last four experiments to obtain the average responses at the respective levels of P, the other effects vanish, as all those effects have an equal number of low and high levels in both the first four and last four experiments. Thus, we can rearrange Table 6.6 in the average responses at low and high levels for any effect. We can similarly show that the impact of the other effects would vanish much in the same way.

Table 6.6: Rearranged design grouping the low level and the high level for P

Trial	Factorial effect						
	P	L	D	PL	PD	LD	PLD
1	−	−	−	+	+	+	−
3	−	+	−	−	+	−	+
5	−	−	+	+	−	−	+
7	−	+	+	−	−	+	−
2	+	−	−	−	−	+	+
4	+	+	−	+	−	−	−
6	+	−	+	−	+	−	−
8	+	+	+	+	+	+	+

A geometric view of the main effects

Rao displayed the 2^3 factorial as a cube plot with the trials at the vertices. Rao identified the trials that contribute to the average of percentage of related substances at the high (+1) level and the low (−1) level for the main effects, P, L, and D. For example, scanning column P from Table 6.6 and the first cube below, we see the trials that contribute to estimating the main effect P.

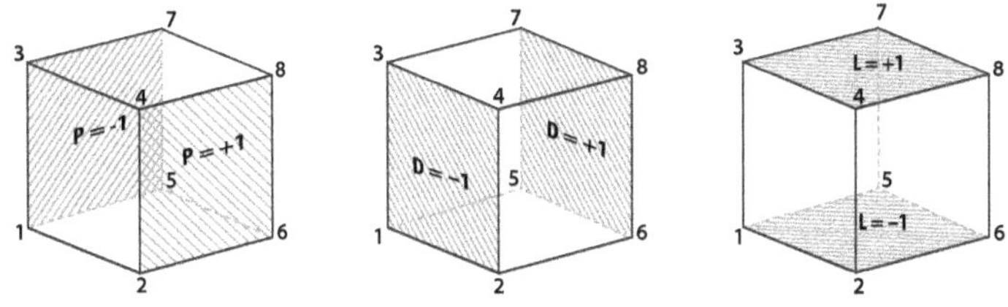

Analyzing the effects

Table 6.7 shows the effect estimates arranged in descending order of magnitude.

Table 6.7: Effect estimates arranged in descending order for the 2^3 factorial design evaluating drug product stability

Effect estimates						
D	P	L	LD	PLD	PL	PD
0.53	0.29	−0.05	0.03	−0.03	0.01	−0.01

The effect estimates given in Table 6.7 do not answer the essential question we are after: which effects significantly contribute to the response? In our specific case, we state the only significant effects are D and P, as their effect estimates are several times bigger in magnitude than the others. The "significance" we seek will be, at best, a relative measure—relative to the magnitude of the other effects. We must compare the effects of D and P against the experimental error to establish statistical significance. We introduced the experimental error in Chapter 5, albeit very briefly. Here we go a little deeper.

Where does the experimental error come from, and what does it mean for our analysis?

Consider the first experiment for which P, L, and D are at their low levels. For this experiment, we obtain the response (percentage of related substances after 6 weeks) value of 0.45. If we run the same experiment one more time (a replication in the design of experiments terminology), can we expect the same response value? Most likely not. Why would the response values from the same experiment replicated twice be different? After all, when we run the same experiment twice, we keep the factors that potentially affect the response at the same level.

But how sure are we of maintaining the levels of the factors at the same level? Issues like measurement system uncertainty may contribute to changes in the levels believed to be the same. Even if we could overlook this issue, might we be overlooking other factors we are aware of yet ignored in the experimentation or factors that we may not even conceive? How do the levels of those factors change from one replication to another? Since we do not record the levels of these additional factors, we combine them all in a single term we call experimental error. Hence, each response includes the potential effect of the chosen experimental factors and their interaction represented by the levels of these effects plus the experimental error composed of an unknown number of effects we are not aware of or decided to ignore. Therefore, we adopt a simple representation of the response, where each response is the sum of the model, which includes all the significant effects and the experimental error, which includes all the insignificant effects.

Response = Model + Error

Following this representation, an effect is deemed significant only relative to the error. Finally, we shall address the concern about all effects in the error term deemed unimportant when discussing the concept of blocking in designing experiments.

Comparing the model to the error compares the signal to the noise, where the signal represents the model, and the noise means the error. This comparison will work as long as we can quantify the error. But how can we quantify something that includes effects we may not know? In experimental work, we generally follow two routes to estimate the amount of experimental error in our data. The first is through replication of experimental runs. The variation we observe in the outcomes of these replications is an excellent measure for our system's level of experimental error. For example, if the responses from a replicated experiment vary wildly, that will indicate a large amount of experimental error and vice versa. However, in general, replication can be a luxury we cannot afford. In such cases we consider the variation in the data that the model does not explain to be reflecting the amount of experimental error, following the additive model above. This second approach generates circular thinking: we judge the model's significance against the error quantified upon establishing the model. The great industrial statistician Cuthbert Daniel proposed a workaround, which is described below.

First, consider the case where none of the effects in the model are significant. In this case, we would expect the response for all experiments to be the same (say a constant), except for the experimental error affecting that experiment. Hence, we would have

Response = Constant + Error

That means we can write the responses as shown in Table 6.8, where e_i represents the experimental error for experiment i.

Table 6.8: The response when no effect is significant

Trial	Factorial effect							Response
	P	L	D	PL	PD	LD	PLD	
1	–	–	–	+	+	+	–	Constant + e_1
3	–	+	–	–	+	–	+	Constant + e_3
5	–	–	+	+	–	–	+	Constant + e_5
7	–	+	+	–	–	+	–	Constant + e_7
2	+	–	–	–	–	+	+	Constant + e_2
4	+	+	–	+	–	–	–	Constant + e_4
6	+	–	+	–	+	–	–	Constant + e_6
8	+	+	+	+	+	+	+	Constant + e_8

Of course, we would not know beforehand there were no significant effects, since that would defeat the purpose of running the experiments in the first place. We can proceed with calculating the effect estimates as described before. For example, the effect estimate for P will simply yield

$$Effect\ of\ P = \frac{(e_2 + e_4 + e_6 + e_8)}{4} - \frac{(e_1 + e_3 + e_5 + e_7)}{4}$$
$$= \frac{1}{4}\left[e_2 + e_4 + e_6 + e_8 - e_1 - e_3 - e_5 - e_7\right]$$

with the constant terms in Table 6.8 washing away. Other effect calculations will yield similar results. The effect estimate will be a summation (with the appropriate signs depending on the effect) of all eight error terms divided by four. The typical approach in modeling in an inferential study assumes the error is normally distributed with mean zero and a constant variance, often referred to as σ^2. We further assume the errors affecting the responses are independent. These assumptions, namely normal distribution, constant variance, and independence of the experimental error, constitute the basis of many inferential studies to determine whether an effect is significant relative to the experimental error.

Following these assumptions, we can show that the effect estimates will follow a normal distribution with mean zero and variance $\sigma^2/2$ if there are no significant effects. We can confirm this through a normal probability plot of the effects. We plot the effect estimates against the theoretical values from the corresponding normal distribution in the normal plot. On that plot, if the effect estimates all fall on a line, meaning the actual effects and theoretical values from a normal distribution match, then the normal distribution assumption is confirmed. Hence, we can conclude that there are no significant effects.

For example, the normal plot in Figure 6.1 shows a hypothetical case where in a 2^3 design none of the seven effects (the main and interaction effects) are significant.

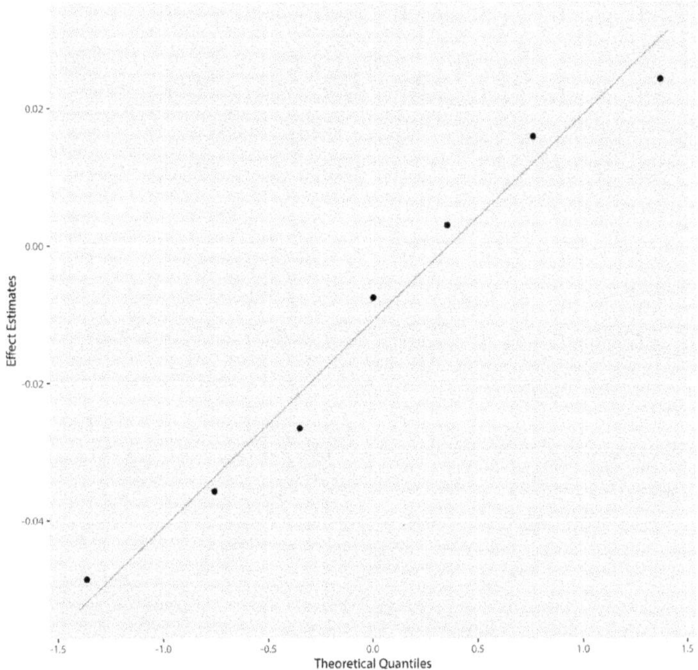

Figure 6.1: A hypothetical case of a normal plot of the effects where no effects are significant.

We can now follow the same analysis for the 2^3 experimental design from Table 6.3. Figure 6.2 is a normal plot of the effect estimates presented in Table 6.7.

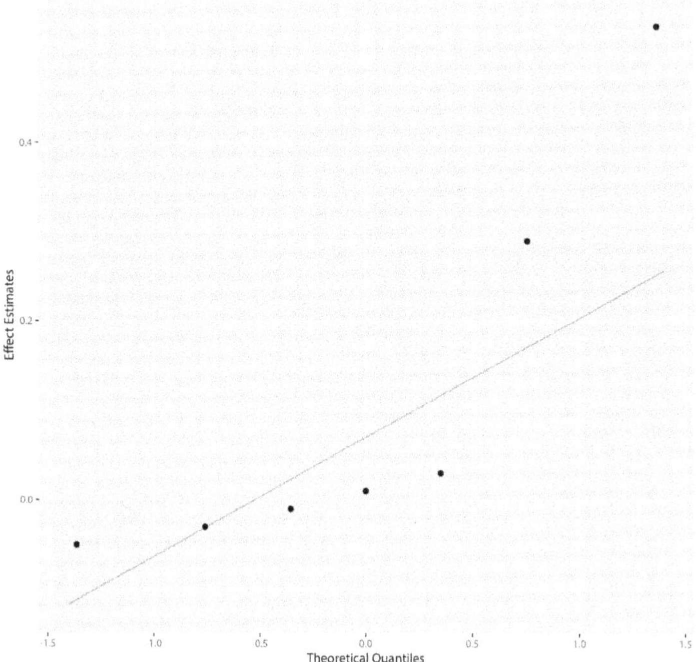

Figure 6.2: The normal plot of the effects from Table 6.7 for the 2^3 factorial design evaluating drug product stability.

We also provide a line attempting to go through all points, but, obviously, it is quite difficult to conclude that the points fall on a line, as the points corresponding to D and P behave quite differently than the others.

Therefore, Figure 6.3 shows a more appropriate line, covering not all but most of the effects. Figure 6.3 helps us conclude the effects follow a normal distribution, except for D and P. Hence, the calculations of these five effects involve some linear combination of normally distributed errors. Therefore, we label D and P only as potentially significant effects. We can perform a more rigorous statistical analysis when the five effects concluded to be insignificant are pooled together as the error component (see "If you wondered," p. 76).

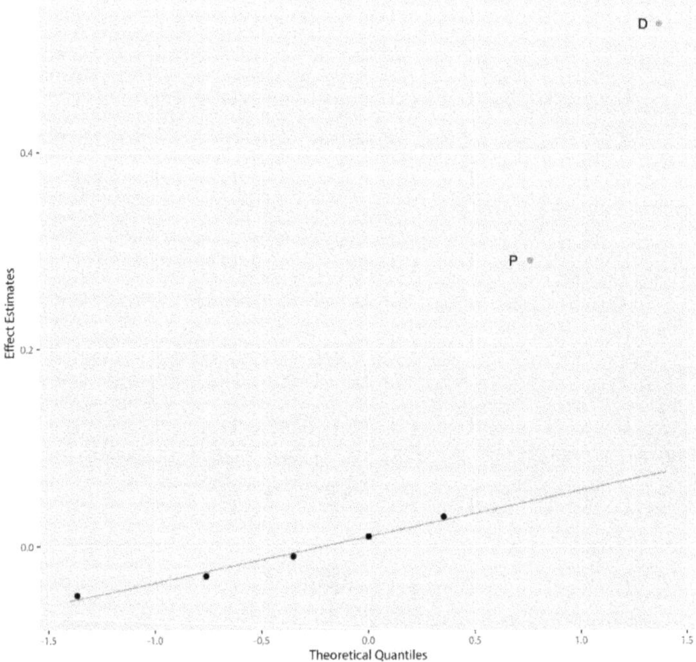

Figure 6.3: The normal plot of the effects for the percentage of related substances %RS showing diluent D, and process P affecting the %RS. The effect estimates are from Table 6.7.

Look at your data

Rao urged Yesim to always look at her data in addition to the statistical analysis. So Yesim used the cube representation to look at their data. On studying the cube, they realized that regardless of the lubricant (L) change, the percentage of related substances did not change more than 0.2%. Recall 0.2% was practically meaningful for these experiments. Therefore, Yesim assumes the lubricant change, L, did not affect the stability. Thus, the 2^3 design becomes a 2^2 factorial for process, P, and diluent, D, which replicated twice, as represented by a square and the tabular display below.

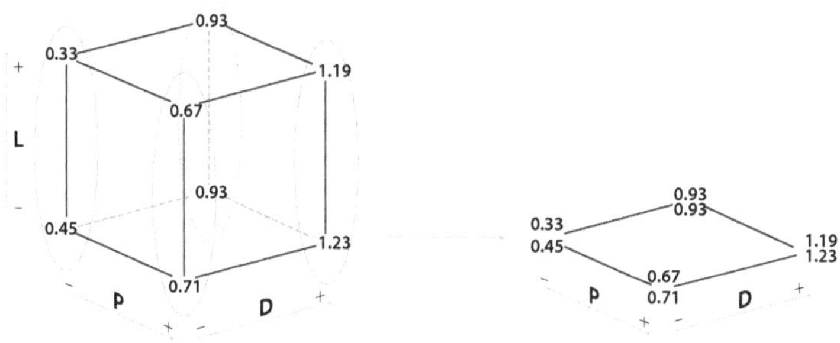

Trials	P	D	%RS
1, 3	–	–	0.45, 0.33
2, 4	+	–	0.71, 0.67
5, 7	–	+	0.93, 0.93
6, 8	+	+	1.23, 1.19

Interpretation

Based on the data and the subsequent analysis, Yesim sees moisture in the process and the presence of lactose negatively influencing the stability of the drug product. Therefore, Yesim decides to consult the organic and physical chemists at the organization to understand the mechanism. In addition, Yesim must consider the maximum dosage strength or drug load per unit tablet or capsule, because there are limitations to the amount of drug that can be accommodated per unit dosage form when using a direct compression process.

What to do next?

Mae suggested testing the drug release profile for Trials 1 and 3 to confirm there are no issues with the drug release from the product. Next, Yesim outlined another set of experiments for a clinical drug product. Using magnesium stearate as the lubricant, they proposed evaluating different strengths with varying proportions of microcrystalline cellulose and starch. Finally, they would conduct stability studies on the drug product in high-density polyethylene bottles.

They decided to investigate how and possibly why moisture affects the drug product stability.

But what if Yesim only had sufficient drug substance to conduct four experiments? The 2^{3-1} design.

During the early stages of product development, there are limits to the available drug substance for product development work. What if Yesim found herself in a situation where the drug substance available is insufficient for eight trials? She will need to decide which trials among those listed in Table 6.3 will give her information on the effect of the excipients on the stability of the drug product.

Yesim asks Rao to help her identify the trials to conduct. Rao introduces Yesim to fractional factorial designs, which offer an option with four trials only. But Rao cautions Yesim that these four experiments are too few for a statistical analysis for significance and may only provide directional guidance.

First, Rao rearranges Table 6.2 based on the minus and the plus signs of the three-factor interaction (Table 6.9). Then, Rao also displays the design geometrically because the vertices of the figures in three dimensions provide excellent experimental designs (see "If you wondered," p. 76).

The four trials (Trials 2, 3, 5, and 8) for which the three-factor interaction, PLD, is always at the high (+1) level constitute the primary half fraction and the other four trials constitute the alternate half fraction (see "If you wondered," p. 76).

Table 6.9: Ordering the eight experiments on the minus and the plus signs of the three-factor interaction, PLD gives two 2^{3-1} designs. Fractional designs are displayed as tetrahedrons in a cube

Trial	Factorial effect							Tetrahedron in a cube
	P	L	D	PL	PD	LD	PLD	
2	+	−	−	−	−	+	+	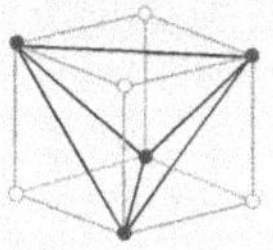
3	−	+	−	−	+	−	+	
5	−	−	+	+	−	−	+	
8	+	+	+	+	+	+	+	
1	−	−	−	+	+	+	−	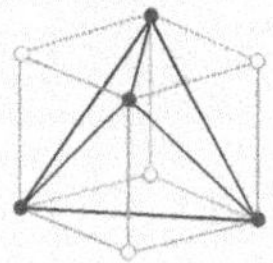
4	+	+	−	+	−	−	−	
6	+	−	+	−	+	−	−	
7	−	+	+	−	−	+	−	

Rao explains that a regular tetrahedron has four vertices. Then, he draws a tetrahedron circumscribed in a cube and shows that the four vertices of the tetrahedron correspond to four trials in a 2^{3-1} design. Note that we write the fractional factorial design (or, to be specific in this case, the half fraction) as 2^{3-1}, which is equal to 2^2. But in factorial designs, 2^2 refers to a design with two factors, both tested at two levels. In this case, we have three factors. Therefore, to avoid potential confusion, we refer to the half fraction design as 2^{3-1}, equivalent to half of a 2^3 design $\left(\frac{2^3}{2}\right)$.

The reduction in the number of runs comes at the price of not being able to estimate PDL. As discussed in the "If you wondered" section on p. 76, main effects and two-factor interactions can no longer be estimated separately, but instead, they will be estimated in pairs as in D and PL, P and DL, and L and PD. We then say that these effects are confounded or aliased. Nonetheless, even in this example, we can use the results for directional guidance. Furthermore, as discussed in the next example, the confounding can be less severe, allowing for a better explanation of the analysis outcome under certain assumptions.

Table 6.10 extracts the primary fraction with responses for a 2^{3-1} experimental arrangement from Table 6.3.

Table 6.10: A 2^{3-1} design to study the effect of the P, L, and D factors on the 6-week stability of a morpholine compound. The design uses four of the eight trials from the 2^3 eight trial design

Trial	P	L	D	%RS
2	+	–	–	0.71
3	–	+	–	0.33
5	–	–	+	0.93
8	+	+	+	1.19

Analysis

Table 6.11 shows the effect estimates for the 2^{3-1} design in Table 6.10. In this case, the main effect estimates from the full factorial in Table 6.7 and Table 6.11 are close. Therefore, we will most likely not be mistaken if we consider factors D and P to be important. Again, however, it is best to consider this small number of experiments as providing directional guidance only because of the confounding.

Table 6.11: Effect estimates arranged in descending order for the 2^{3-1} design in Table 6.10

Effect estimates		
D	P	L
0.54	0.32	-0.06

A brief detour on planning of experiments

The key to success in experimentation is good planning and careful preparation.

—Søren Bisgaard, 1998

We use a problem, constraints, resources, design (PCRD) framework when planning experiments. Thus we ask ourselves a series of what, why, how, when, which, and where questions (Table 6.12). By going through these questions, we slow down our thinking when considering a multifactorial experiment or problem. The experimental design decision comes last because the design should fit the situation. Thus, we recommend thinking through the questions for multifactorial experimentation. We do not recommend going through all the questions for minor issues or for those where the subject matter expert knows the two or three best experiments to conduct. The PCRD framework should not be a bureaucratic chore, and the questions in Table 6.12 are not prescriptive. The framework reflects the need to know the basics we learn in school: our objective, the expected outcome, and how we measure the output.

Identifying an initial formulation and the manufacturing method

Yesim, the formulator, and Mae, the analyst, had to develop a dosage form for a small molecule. Mae's study showed the compound could hydrolyze in aqueous media and was more stable at pH<5. Yesim knew they had the drug substance to complete ten experiments at a small scale, and Mae agreed to support the analysis. They approached Rao for his statistical expertise regarding the planning of experiments.[1] Rao suggested they review the PCRD framework (Table 6.12).

Table 6.12: Output from the experimental planning meeting

Problem			
	Question	Answer	Comments
What	What is the goal of our experiment?	Identify the excipients and method of manufacture.	Identify the qualitative formulation and a method of manufacture.
What	What are we trying to answer?	Are there chemical incompatibilities between the drug substance and excipients?	None.
Why	Why is it important to answer?	We do not want to include excipient incompatible with the drug substance because it will reduce the shelf life of the drug product and could produce undesired degradants.	We are identifying a qualitative formulation.

1 Statisticians have developed experimental design thinking to plan experiments for a better outcome. Even with the availability of the software that enables experimenters to design and analyze experiments without consulting a statistician it is good practice to review the planning questions.

Problem			
	Question	Answer	Comments
What	What is the next action if we answer the question?	We will include the compatible excipients from these experiments and continue experimenting with excipients from other categories. We have to identify the process and evaluate process parameters.	We need to define the qualitative and quantitative formulation for the clinical drug product.
How	How many factors do we want to study?	Four.	Process, lubricant, diluent, and disintegrant.
How	How many levels of each factor do we want to include?	Two.	See Table 6.3.
How	How many responses might we measure?	Assay, percentage of related substances, and appearance.	Need to have <1.5% total degradation and less than 0.4% individual for this study.

Constraints			
	Questions	Answers	Comments
Which	Which factors will not be studied?	Process parameters. The particle size of the drug substance or the excipients.	Evaluate at the next set of trials.
Which	Which factors will be held constant?	Process parameters, same operators, analytical testing parameters.	We are at the first step of identifying a process and equipment train and formulation components.
What	What are the uncontrollable factors? Example: environmental factors (temperature, humidity, pressure), operator to operator variability, time, measurement variability.	Operate at ambient temperature and humidity based on the facilities. Use available equipment for the process.	Record the room temperature and humidity in the room.

Constraints			
	Questions	Answers	Comments
What	Are there limits to conducting the experiments in the prescribed order? (Examples are equipment changes, material availability, bulk processing, measuring a batch of samples at a time.)	There are no constraints for these experiments.	There is no need for blocking in these experiments.
What	What is our proposed experimental design?	A 2^{4-1} fractional factorial.	Eight runs.
What	What is our approach to statistical analysis?	Data tables, plots, numerical analysis.	Always look at the data.
What	Timeline	Three months.	It cannot exceed four months.
What	Anticipated problems.	Drug substance shortage, scheduling issues, instrument downtime.	Keep track and plan 2 weeks ahead.

Resources			
	Question	Answer	Comments
Who	People	Jolene and Sam from operations, Yesim and Billie from development, Mae and Aretha from analytical, and Rao from the statistical group.	None.
How Much	Budget	Internal budget.	See Appendix A for using experimental design to estimate a budget.
Where	Location	East wing facility of Bldg. A.	
When	Timeline	End by August 2021.	

Design			
	Question	Answer	Comments
How	Do we need exploratory runs?	The experimentation and preparation techniques are not new.	No exploratory run is needed.
How	How many experiments or trials can we conduct?	We have the drug substance for nine experiments.	Please note the color of the drug substance in the records.
How	How many qualitative factors?	Four.	None.
How	How many quantitative factors?	None.	None.
What	What is the estimate of the measurement error?	HPLC analysis of related substances: ±0.5% or even ±1%.	We will refine the methods and complete robustness studies as the development continues into Phase 3 clinical trials.
What	What is the current subject matter knowledge?	Hydrolysis could occur. We are uncertain about the interaction between the excipients and the amine group. The supply chain does not prefer novel excipients. The primary response variable is percentage of related substances at this stage.	Yesim and Mae will have to understand the mechanisms or consult the chemists. It may occur in parallel if product development can continue without knowing the cause.

The 2^{4-1} design

The number of experiments in a two-level factorial for three factors is eight (2^3), for four factors is 16 (2^4), and for five factors is 32 (2^5). The number of experiments in a two-level full factorial design increases considerably with the number of factors. Usually, we have enough drug substance or time, personnel, and equipment needed for eight to 24 experiments at the early stages. Fractional factorial designs address this problem by having a smaller number of runs while still providing reasonable estimates. But as stated before, we lose information, which results in less clarity in our analysis (also see "If you wondered," p. 76).

We again show the fractional factorial design idea with an eight-run design to evaluate four factors. We consider the half fraction of a 2^4 design, a 2^{4-1} fractional factorial, which is a half fraction because we have $\frac{2^4}{2} = 8$ trials.

We can, in this case, employ the same methodology we used in the case of the 2^{3-1} design. We can write the 2^4 full factorial design matrix, consider the column for the fourth-order interaction effect, then select the eight runs for which this effect is at the high level, hence sacrificing this effect and picking the principal fraction. An alternative approach to generating this design is the following. We start with the 2^3 design given in Table 6.2. Now assume that Yesim wants to include a fourth factor, T, in this design. For a given trial, all they need is to know at which level they should test the factor T. They can use any of the seven columns in Table 6.2 for that purpose, as they will all provide the necessary levels to test factor T. However, we now know this implies the main effect T is confounded with that particular effect. At this point, we should ask which of the seven effects in Table 6.2 is less likely to be significant. The answer is, once again, the PLD interaction. The design for the main effects only is given in Table 6.13. We can show that the resulting confounding (alias) pattern is

Effect	Aliased with
P	LDT
L	PDT
D	PLT
T	PLD
PL	DT
PD	LT
LD	PT

Yesim has confounded the four main effects with the three-factor interactions by choosing a half fraction. Yet, she can estimate these main effects clearly if we assume the three-factor interactions are negligible. For example, suppose PLD interaction is indeed negligible. In that case, the effect calculation corresponding to the sum of T and PLD will only refer to T. This will also be the case for other main effects. However, Yesim cannot estimate the PL, PD, and LD interactions independently of DT, LT, and PT, respectively. In general, we choose the fractional factorial, so the main effect estimates are, as far as possible, confounded with higher-order effects, which are expected to be negligible.

Experimental data

Table 6.13 shows the results of the planned experiments.

Table 6.13: A 2^{4-1} experimental design for studying excipient compatibility and identifying the drug product manufacturing method. Column T is a product of P, L, and D

Trial	Order	P	L	D	T	%RS
1	2	–	–	–	–	1.94
2	5	+	–	–	+	0.58
3	4	–	+	–	+	7.40
4	1	+	+	–	–	3.18
5	7	–	–	+	+	1.38
6	8	+	–	+	–	0.42
7	6	–	+	+	–	7.26
8	3	+	+	+	+	2.72
	–	WG	SA	M/S	PVP XL	
	+	DC	MS	L/S	CCS	

P: process; L: lubricant; D: diluent; T: disintegrant
WG: wet granulation; DC: direct compression
SA: stearic acid; MS: magnesium stearate
M/S: microcrystalline cellulose/pregelatinized starch (70:30)
L/S: lactose/pregelatinized starch (80:20)
PVPXL: polynvinypyrrolidone XL; CCS: croscarmellose sodium
%RS: percentage of related substances after 6 weeks

Analysis

We start the data analysis with the normal plot of the effects shown in Figure 6.4.

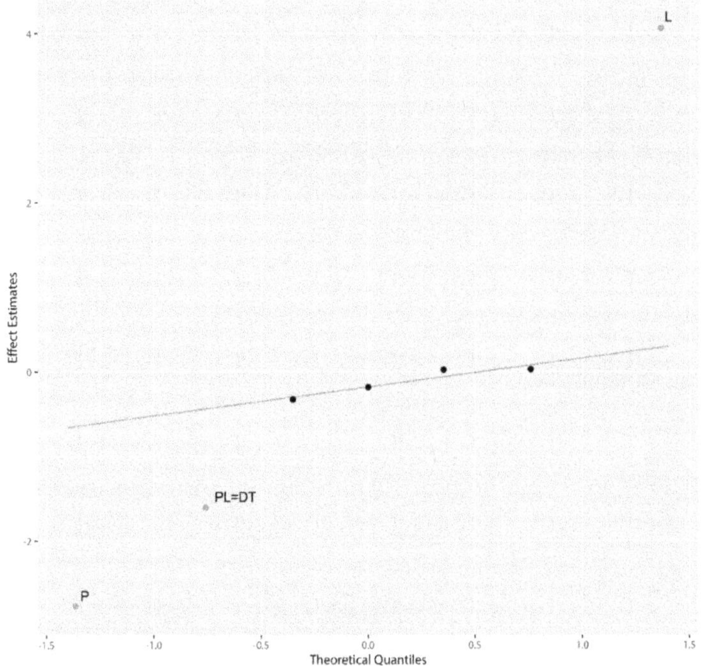

Figure 6.4: The normal plot of the effects for the percentage of related substances %RS showing how the process P, lubricant L, and the interaction between P and L (and/or disintegrant D and lubricant L) affect the %RS.

From Figure 6.4 the main effects of P and L seem significant. We know that P and L are confounded with LDT and PDT, respectively. Hence, the effect calculation associated with P and L corresponds to P + LDT and L + PDT, respectively. However, if we assume that third- and higher-order interactions are negligible, in that case, we can simply conclude that the main effects of P and L are estimated to be free from confounding. The third significant effect corresponds to the confounded pair of PL and DT interactions. In general, there is no way for us to know if these effects are significant. However, we choose the simplest explanation for an occurrence using Occam's razor. Since the main effects of P and L appear significant in this situation, it is more likely that the PL interaction than the DT interaction is significant. We tentatively infer that P, L, and PL effects are significant. For the statistical analysis of this example, please refer to the supplemental material on the book's website.

Look at your data

Once Rao's analysis identified P, L, and PL as significant effects through statistical analysis, Yesim realized the design projects into a replicated 2^2 design. Using only the P and L columns, they rearranged their data from Table 6.13 in descending order and drew a square plot representing a 2^2 design.

Trial	Order	P	L	%RS
3	4	–	+	7.40
7	6	–	+	7.26
4	1	+	+	3.18
8	3	+	+	2.72
1	2	–	–	1.94
5	7	–	–	1.38
2	5	+	–	0.58
6	8	+	–	0.42
	–	WG	SA	
	+	DC	MS	

A projected 2^2 design

P: process; WG: wet granulation; DC: direct compression;
L: lubricant; SA: stearic acid; MS: magnesium stearate

Interpretation

The square plot suggests that Yesim may consider using the direct compression process and stearic acid as the lubricant in the future. In addition, Yesim will use a mixture of lactose anhydrous and pregelatinized starch to enable a compressible tablet dosage form. They elected to use croscarmellose sodium in future trials because it was commonly available within their supply chain.

The wet granulation process contributed to the possible hydrolysis, and the interaction shown in Figure 6.5 between the process and lubricant, specifically wet granulation and magnesium stearate, indicated a potential role of the microenvironmental pH in degradation. Mae's earlier data showing the compound could hydrolyze in aqueous media and was more stable at pH<5 is significant here. However, Mae and Yesim questioned the significant degradation observed when using magnesium stearate as a lubricant in the direct compression process. The hypothesis was the storage condition contributed to this effect.

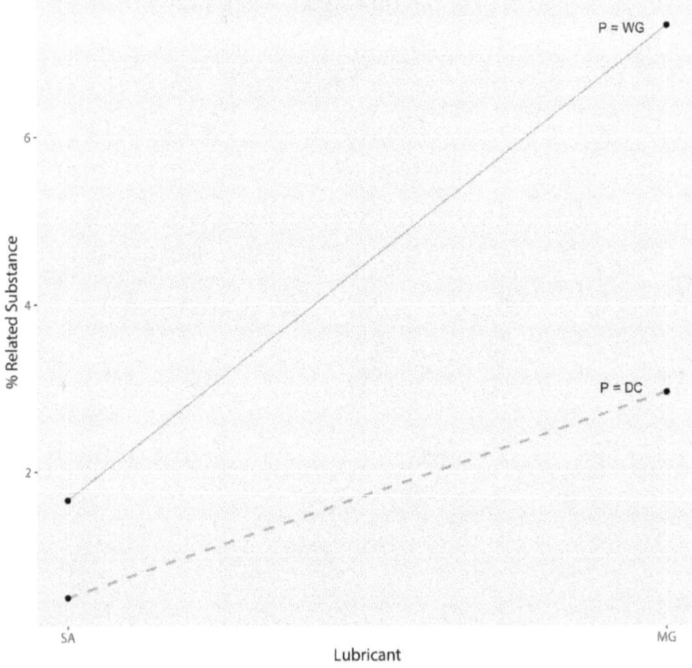

Figure 6.5: The plot indicates a potential interaction between the lubricant L and process P. SA is stearic acid, MG is magnesium stearate, WG is wet granulation, and DC is direct compression.

What to do next?

If the dose needed for clinical studies was high and the percentage of drug loading per tablet was too high, Yesim must explore a roller compaction process. They decided to explore the particle size of the drug substance, the percentage of excipients, and some initial process parameters in the next series of experiments.

If you wondered

A more rigorous statistical analysis for the 2^3 experiment at the beginning of the chapter

In the example of the 2^3 design, we first tentatively identify the main effects of P and D as significant effects. Hence, these two effects constitute our model. The leftover five effects are simply deemed not significant and therefore dropped from the model. But where do they go? Recall we described the response in terms of the model, and the error as representing all of the insignificant factors combined. In that sense, it is natural to think the effects that are deemed insignificant would go to the error. We should also remember that when we declare significance, it is always relative to the error. An effect can only be significant if its influence on the response is large compared to the error. In this context, we compare the variation caused by the effect (or the model) relative to the variation caused by the error. We compare the so-called mean squares of the effect (or the model) to the mean squares of the error. If that ratio (and hence the variation caused by the effect over the variation caused by the error) is large enough, we deem the effect significant. But how large is large enough? While we can use some rules of thumb, a rigorous approach is based on the probability distribution of the ratio given by the F-distribution, which is named after R. A. Fisher, the father of modern statistics. The F-distribution is valid under the assumptions that the errors are independent, identically distributed with normal distribution with mean 0 and a constant variance. We should confirm the validity of these assumptions through the residual analysis.

Below is an analysis of variance (ANOVA) table for the model with only P and D main effects. We can conclude the effects are significant at a 5% significance level since the p-values are less than 0.05. Recall, in this case, the magnitude of the effect is also practically meaningful. For a more technical and detailed discussion of the statistical analysis of experimental data, we refer readers to Box, Hunter, and Hunter (2005).

	Sum of Squares	Degrees of Freedom	Mean Squares	F-ratio	*p*-value
P	0.1682	1	0.1682	93.44	0.0002
D	0.5618	1	0.5618	312.11	$\sim 10^{-5}$
Error	0.0090	5	0.0018		
Total	0.7390	7			

Why is the test of significance important?

The significance test helps us avoid jumping to conclusions on the slightest evidence when common variation in our experiments may explain an effect. Granted, experimenters may not be interested in significance testing but want to know if the difference between the treatments and their magnitude is practically important. Nevertheless, when possible, it is a good practice for the experimenter to define a meaningful difference.

Significance testing of the effects using the *p*-values is based on the assumptions of the experimental error we discussed in this chapter. Recall that we assume the experimental error to be independent and normally distributed with a constant variance. Violations in any of these assumptions will affect our conclusions from the ANOVA. Therefore, we should never end any statistical analysis of the experimental data with the ANOVA but follow it by confirming the assumptions imposed on the experimental error. But how can we confirm these assumptions since we do not know the experimental error?

We introduced the experimental error to represent all effects that are not significant and hence not included in the model. That implies that if we knew the true model, we could subtract the model from the response to obtain the experimental error. But we need to find out the true model too. All we have is an estimate of the true model through the estimates of the significant effects. But suppose that estimate is "good" enough. In that case, we can subtract the estimated model (also called the fitted values) from the response to obtain the so-called residuals, which mimic the experimental error and hence have similar characteristics. Therefore, if the model is estimated correctly, the residuals should be independent and normally distributed with a constant variance. While there are some rigorous tests we can employ, we would often resort to visual tools, as in normal probability plotting of the residuals for normality check, plotting the residuals against the fitted values and factor levels for checking the constant variance assumption or plotting the residuals against the run order of the trials for checking the independence assumption. All these efforts constitute the so-called residual analysis. We provide the residual analysis of this case on the book's website. (datatodecision.org.)

Geometric representation of two-level designs

Regular polyhedra often appear in nature, science, engineering, sports, and experimental designs:

- At the crystallization stage in drug substance manufacturing, randomly organized molecules in a fluid come together to form an ordered three-dimensional molecular array with a periodic repeating pattern.
- Crystals have their atoms arranged in a regular grid consisting of tetrahedra, cubes, and octahedra.
- Tetrahedra and octahedra shapes help construct roofs and bridges because they are rigid and stable.
- The most famous polyhedron in the world is the truncated icosahedron: it is the shape of a soccer ball.

- The vertices of regular figures in three dimensions provide excellent experimental designs. The table below provides a geometrical view of some basic two-level designs.

Geometric shape		Design*	Number of trials
Line		1^2	2
Square	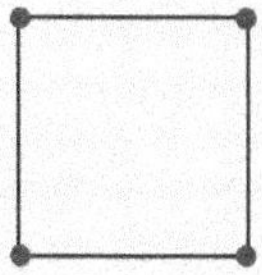	2^2	4
Cube	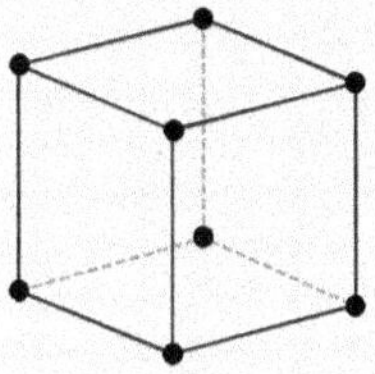	2^3	8
Tetrahedron in a cube	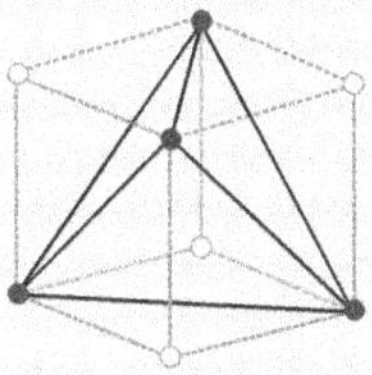	2^{3-1}	4
Tetrahedron in a cube	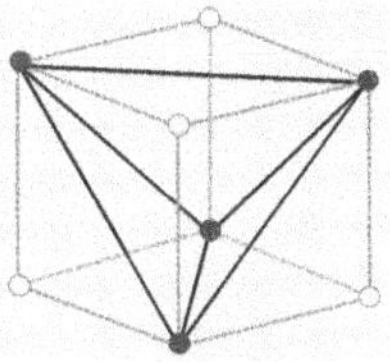	Alternate 2^{3-1}	4
Obtuse wedge as a bisected regular tetrahedron	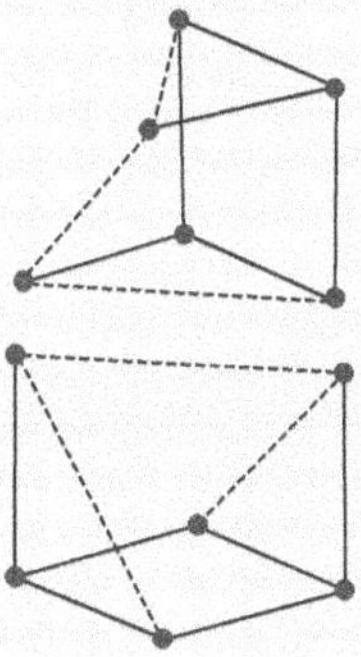	$3\ (2^{3-2})$	6

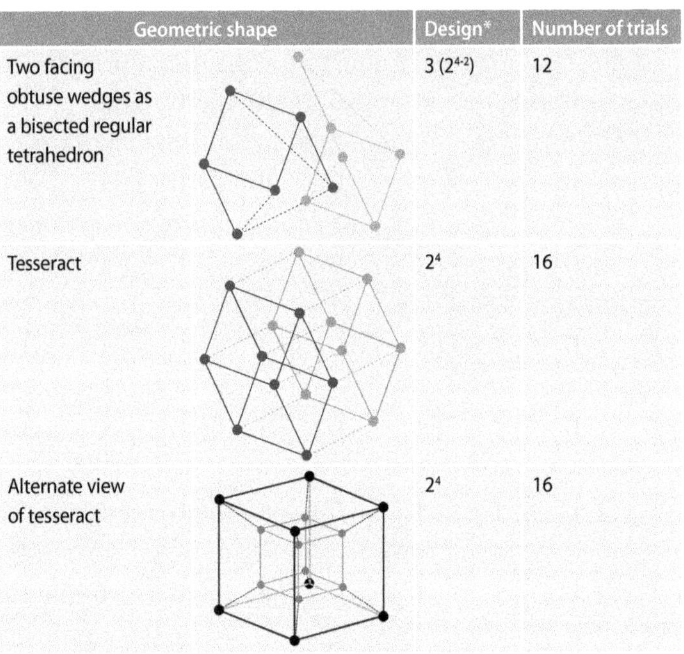

Geometric shape		Design*	Number of trials
Two facing obtuse wedges as a bisected regular tetrahedron		$3\ (2^{4-2})$	12
Tesseract		2^4	16
Alternate view of tesseract		2^4	16

*The base represents the level, and the first superscript number represents the number of factors.

Why does Rao propose the 2^{3-1} designs?

Let's go back to the original premise: We could only afford four experiments but the full factorial, in this case, would require eight experiments. We can show 70 different ways of picking four (without any replications) out of the eight experiments given in Table 6.1. For example, the first four trials in Table 6.1 are such a potential set. Or the first three trials plus the fifth, first three trials plus the sixth, etc. At any rate, it is difficult to sift through 70 different sets to find the right set of four experiments. So, we start putting some conditions on the final set of experiments we pick.

Based on our previous explanation of the vanishing of the other effects (Table 6.6), a reasonable and somewhat intuitive approach is to select four experiments with an equal number of low and high levels for each effect during the calculation of an effect. With this condition, the number of sets of experiments to consider reduces to 14 from 70. Furthermore, we need to consider only seven sets of four experiments for a group complying with this condition. A complementary set consisting of the four leftover experiments will also automatically adhere to the condition, as all columns in Table 6.1 have an equal number of pluses and minuses.

Consider the set of four trials (Trials 2, 4, 6, and 8) in the table below together with the complementary (leftover) trials. For these four trials (as well as the complementary set), all effects have an equal number of pluses and minuses except for the effect of P. This means that we can estimate all effects except for P because, to assess an effect, we should test it at different levels. The first consequence of running fewer trials is less information because we cannot expect to gain the same amount of information from a system we are investigating when we use a fraction of a complete factorial design. By choosing to run fewer trials, we also accept that we will not be able to estimate all effects, as we would using a full factorial design. In the case of the design in Table below, it is apparent that the effect that is being sacrificed is the main effect of factor P.

A possible half fraction (and its complementary half fraction) for a 2^3 design is shown below.

Trial	Factorial effect						
	P	L	D	PL	PD	LD	PLD
2	+	–	–	–	–	+	+
4	+	+	–	+	–	–	–
6	+	–	+	–	+	–	–
8	+	+	+	+	+	+	+
1	–	–	–	+	+	+	–
3	–	+	–	–	+	–	+
5	–	–	+	+	–	–	+
7	–	+	+	–	–	+	–

We often view the likelihood of the significance of the effects being highest for the main effects followed by the second-order interaction effects, third-order interaction effects, and so on. In that regard, sacrificing a main effect seems somewhat extreme in the pursuit of reducing the number of runs by half. Following the above hierarchy, if we were to sacrifice an effect, the most reasonable choice appears to be the highest-order interaction, which is the PLD interaction effect in this case. Trials 2, 3, 5, and 8 for which PLD interaction effect is always at the high level, form the desired half fraction as shown in the table below. The table also shows the complementary set of Trials 1, 4, 6, and 7, when PLD is at a low level. Both groups are the most viable choices following the requirement of sacrificing an effect. Conventionally, the first set for which the PLD interaction is at a high level is considered the primary fraction.

The primary half fraction (and its complementary half fraction) of a 2^3 design when we sacrifice the PLD interaction effect is shown below.

Trial	Factorial effect						
	P	L	D	PL	PD	LD	PLD
2	+	–	–	–	–	+	+
3	–	+	–	–	+	–	+
5	–	–	+	+	–	–	+
8	+	+	+	+	+	+	+
1	–	–	–	+	+	+	–
4	+	+	–	+	–	–	–
6	+	–	+	–	+	–	–
7	–	+	+	–	–	+	–

However, is this the only price we bear when going from eight experiments to only four? For this gain, we only lose the ability to estimate PLD interaction, which may as well be assumed insignificant as it is unlikely that the three factors interact and meaningfully affect the response. However, we make this assumption in many situations, and fractional factorial designs primarily rely on the significance of a few low-order effects. Hence, we may inadvertently conclude that we have gained more than we have lost.

We can now look solely at the primary fraction of the 2^{3-1} design in the table below.

Trial	Factorial Effect						
	P	L	D	PL	PD	LD	PLD
2	+	–	–	–	–	+	+
3	–	+	–	–	+	–	+
5	–	–	+	+	–	–	+
8	+	+	+	+	+	+	+

For illustration purposes, consider the effect estimation for D. Following the arguments above, we can estimate the main effect of D by comparing the average response for Trials 5 and 8 with the average response for Trials 2 and 3. D is at the high level for Trials 5 and 8 and at the low level for Trials 2 and 3. Thus, any significant difference we see in these averages should be due to a change in the levels of D. Yet it is also striking to observe that the PL interaction effect follows precisely the same pattern for those averages. For Trials 5 and 8, the PL interaction effect is at the high level, whereas it is at the low level for Trials 2 and 3. This raises the possibility that either the main effect of D, the interaction effect PL, or both explain the significant difference between the average responses for Trials 5 and 8 on the one hand and 2 and 3 on the other. The effect calculation as the difference of these averages will simply refer to the sum of the main effect of D and the interaction effect PL, and there is no way for us to distinguish these two effects. They are said to be "confounded" or "aliased." In the full factorial case, we could estimate the effects of D and PL separately from each other. However, the estimation of one effect had nothing to do with another effect because of the design's orthogonality. In the half fraction, we simply lost the ability to estimate the effects independently. Upon a second look at the previous table, we observe a similar situation for P and DL, and L and PD. The second unfortunate consequence of using a half fraction rather than the full factorial is confounding.

In summary, by reducing the number of runs by half, we inadvertently give up on both:

1. estimating the effect of PDL, and
2. estimating D and PL, P and DL, and L and PD separately.

For the reason we have discussed, the first consequence is somewhat acceptable. However, the second consequence could seriously impair our analysis as potentially both the main effect and a second-order interaction as in D and PL, or just one of these effects, could significantly affect the response. Thus, there is no way for us to offer a clear conclusion. However, this should not deter anyone from using fractional factorials in general.

NOTES

Box, G.E.P, Hunter, W.G., and Hunter, J.S. in their 2005 book *Statistics for Experimenters: Design, Innovation, and Discovery*. NY: Wiley, state, "It is not unusual for a well-designed experiment to analyze itself." Our analysis is often simplified when we follow a process (with subject matter knowledge) in planning and designing the experiments as outlined in this chapter.

Most experimenters can benefit from a careful reading of Daniel, C. (1976). *Applications of Statistics to Industrial Experimentation*. NY: Wiley. The book's rather terse writing style covers several topics not included in statistical textbooks.

In inferential studies, we aim to make inferences (conclude) beyond the available data. In the book, we try to make conclusions using the available data about the significance of the factor's influence on the response. In that sense, many of the analyses we employ in this book will fall into the inferential category. Refer to Box, Hunter, and Hunter (2005) for further illustrations of such studies and the statistical analyses involved.

Definitive screening designs (DSD) have been proposed as alternatives to two-level fractional factorial designs. DSDs are three-level designs allowing the experimenter to study the effects of many factors in a small number of experiments. The experimenter can study second-order quadratic effects.

The analysis stage is more complex since DSDs are often fully saturated designs, and interactions and quadratic terms are partially confounded.

The originator of experimental design, R.A. Fisher, stated the principles of experimental design in his seminal 1926 paper* as follows:

- Blocks
- Random arrangement
- Replication
- Complex experimentation
- Making comparisons within and between factors
- Conclusions are drawn on a wider inductive basis
- Interactions
- Confounding

*Fisher, R.A. (1926). The arrangement of field experiments. *Journal of the Ministry of Agriculture of Great Britain* 33: 503–513.

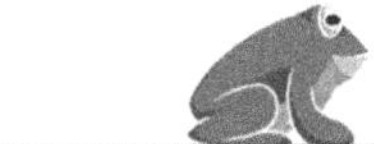

Product development is a continuous dialogue between thought and doing, idea and prototype, and possible and achievable.

7

How Does Experimental Design Enable Formulation Development?

Drug products that enable early phase clinical programs include

- A drug in a capsule or powder in a bottle is a quick approach to dosing subjects in Phase 1 trials. However, this approach may not suit drugs with high doses and poor solubility characteristics.
- A formulated drug product needs a longer time for development, analytical characterization, stability, and manufacturing. However, the formulation could address dose, solubility, and manufacturing issues. Later-phase clinical studies may use the early clinical drug product without changing the product composition. The information helpful to design the drug product includes safety and dose ranging from preclinical studies, the solubility of the drug substance in an aqueous medium, pH buffers and solvents, available physical and chemical

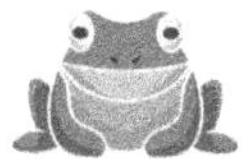

stability of the drug substance, and knowing if the drug must be delivered to a particular gastrointestinal site.

Initial studies in formulation development include identifying the combination of excipients for the dosage form. Knowing the influence of excipient on the stability and performance of the drug product is essential in designing and developing a good drug product. Excipients include diluents, binders, disintegrants, antioxidants, acidifying/alkalizing agents, plasticizers, coating agents, and lubricants. The combination and concentration of the excipients depend on their functionality in the drug product.

The combination of various excipients is tested effectively in an experimental design matrix. The responses are in vitro dosage form performance and stability. Responses include physical and chemical testing.

Should we develop a capsule or a tablet?

Medbox Therapeutics acquired a molecule (FN8324) from Fisson Biotherapeutics that completed Phase 1 trials. Phase 1 trials used the drug substance in a capsule. Medbox wanted to prepare for the Phase 2 clinical study. The project team preferred a tablet dosage form for Phase 2 trials as a potential registration study. On reviewing the physical and chemical characteristics, the CMC team wanted to conduct preliminary studies before developing a tablet dosage form. The drug substances characterization indicated the possibility of a change in the polymorph under physical stress.

Yesim from the product development department reviewed the data package from Fisson Biotherapeutics and identified the available information.

- An indication the drug substance form could be affected under moderate physical stress.

- The drug substance was highly soluble with a pH-independent solubility profile.
- The permeability was high in ex vivo experiments.
- The excipient compatibility studies indicated one related substance of interest. The study also gave a list of diluents, disintegrants, and lubricants for a formulated drug product.
- Yesim decided to formulate a tablet, fill the formulation blends in a capsule, and evaluate the chemical stability.

Yesim decided which excipients should be evaluated in capsule and tablet dosage forms. She knew of the 2^3 experimental designs but asked Rao the statistician about using half of the powder blend from an experiment for capsules and the other half for tablets. Rao expressed concern about Yesim's plans, pointing out that mistakes in weighing the excipients, the speed with which the operators ran the blender, or the total number of revolutions during the preparation of a particular blend would affect the outcome for both the tablet and capsule using that blend. Earlier chapters discussed mitigating such an issue by running the experiments in random order (randomization).

Considering the dosage form (capsule or tablet) as the fourth factor, Rao argued they should execute a 2^4 experimental design in random order. He pointed out that if any unforeseen problems were to happen during the preparation of the blend, only the experiment with the corresponding drug delivery dosage form (capsule or tablet) would be affected.

The truth is both Yesim and Rao were correct in their thinking. Classically trained Rao wanted to execute the experiments in random order rather than systematically to ensure that each experiment would have the same risk of being affected by an unforeseen problem as reflected in the experimental error. Running the experiments in random order satisfies an assumption on which the statistical ANOVA is based. Yesim's plan is more practical, because a completely randomized 2^4 design would require her to prepare 16 different powder blends. Each trial requires more drug substance, personnel, facility, and equipment time. A more convenient approach is to prepare eight different powder blends based on the three factors affecting the blend and split each formulated blend into two portions for the tablet and capsule dosage forms.

Convenience in terms of physical or economic constraints typically takes precedence in experimentation. Complete randomization can be considered utopian in an industrial investigation. In tests such as Yesim and Rao were planning, factors that are easier to change (dosage form) are considered separately from the harder-to-change factors (diluent, disintegrant, lubricant). Thus, randomization is restricted for a given combination of harder-to-change factors while labs run multiple experiments for easier-to-change factors. The resulting designs are called split-plot designs, as they were initially used in agricultural experimentation. A plot of land is split into smaller plots, called whole plots, for the hard-to-apply factors, and each whole plot is further divided into so-called subplots for the easy-to-apply factors. In our example, the eight powder blends representing the whole plot are executed in random order. The dosage form (capsule or tablet) constitutes the subplots within a whole plot. These subplots are run in random order for a given powder blend. More specifically, in this case, a powder blend is split into two portions and used for either capsules or tablets.

This convenience in running split-plot experiments comes at a cost. The most obvious concern is the issue of an error in the preparation of a powder blend affecting not just one but two experiments (subplots), creating a correlation among the responses belonging to the subplots from the same whole plot. Such concerns complicate the analysis of experimental results.

Experimental Data

Yesim carried out the experiments to evaluate the effect of excipients on the stability of the compound FN8324. The results, shown in Table 7.1, are percentage of related substances after storing the product in high-density polyethylene bottles at 50°C/80%RH for 8 weeks. The process was a simple dry blend and had no issues during encapsulation or compression to a tablet. Other dosage form characteristics, including appearance, disintegration, dissolution, tablet hardness, and tablet friability, were acceptable.

Table 7.1: A $2^3 \times 2^1$ split-plot design to evaluate the diluent ratios, disintegrant, and lubricant type effect on FN8324 capsule and tablet stability stored at 50°C/80%RH for 8 weeks

Trial	Order	R	D	L	F capsule	F tablet
					%RS	%RS
1	6	–	–	–	0.51	0.65
2	1	+	–	–	0.42	0.45
3	7	–	+	–	0.20	0.23
4	2	+	+	–	0.24	0.19
5	5	–	–	+	0.41	0.68
6	3	+	–	+	0.36	0.46
7	4	–	+	+	0.00	0.14
8	8	+	+	+	0.00	0.02
	–	80:20	PVPXL	SSF		
	+	60:40	CCS	MS		

R: ratio of microcrystalline cellulose to pregelatinized starch, MCC: PS
D: disintegrant type. PVPXL: crosslinked polyvinylpyrrolidone; CCS: croscarmellose sodium
L: lubricant type. SSF: sodium stearyl fumarate; MS: magnesium stearate
F: dosage form: capsule or tablet
%RS: percentage of related substances. 0.00 indicates below the limit of quantitation.

Analysis

Before Rao performed the analysis, he first visualized the data using the trellis plot in Figure 7.1. These trellis plots are executed as facet plots in the ggplot2 package in R. It displays the data arranged so that the rows represent different levels of the subplot factor (F, the dosage form). The columns represent different levels of two whole-plot factors (D, disintegrant type, and L, lubricant type). The x-axis (R, ratio of microcrystalline cellulose to pregelatinized starch) represents a whole-plot factor.

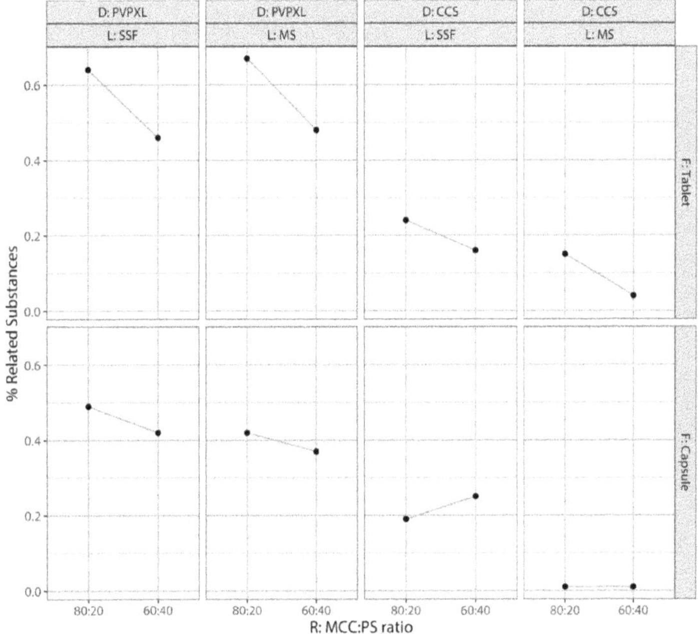

Figure 7.1: The trellis plot shows the effect of disintegrant on the percentage of related substances %RS for FN8324 capsules and tablets stored at 50°C/80%RH for 8 weeks.

Figure 7.1 shows a higher percentage of related substances for disintegrant PVPXL than for CCS. There is no discernable difference between the capsule and tablet dosage forms.

Rao did additional analysis beyond the visualization provided by the trellis plots. The statistical analysis of split-plot designs requires some care since these designs violate complete randomization of the experimental runs for the standard analysis approach using ANOVA. This requirement follows from the assumption of the independence of the errors. For the traditional analysis approach to work, we need to assume that the experimental error affecting one run is independent of the experimental error affecting another run. However, in a split-plot design, an error in a whole plot inevitably affects all subplots run within that whole plot. Suppose Yesim made a mistake in the ratio of microcrystalline cellulose to pregelatinized starch in the first trial. Such an error would affect both dosage forms since she would have used the same powder blend (produced with that mistake) for the capsule and tablet dosage forms In split-plot designs, we run experiments (subplots) within experiments (whole plots), which implies splitting the error into two parts: the whole plot-to-whole plot error and, within a whole plot, a subplot-to-subplot error. The proper analysis needs to take this double error structure into account.

Most statistical analysis examples for split-plot designs involve replicated designs and obtaining the error variance estimations for both errors through the replications. There are only a few proposed methods available for unreplicated split-plot plans. We will show the extension of the approach based on the normal plot of the effects as in the case of unreplicated factorial designs in Chapter 6. It may be tempting to calculate all effects and then have the normal plot of the effects as in Chapter 6. However, due to the double error structure of the split-plot designs, this can be misleading. As shown in the following discussions, the usual effect calculations will imply that we can classify the effects into two groups depending on which errors are present in the calculations.

Table 7.2: The whole plots and the subplots

Trial	WP	SP	R	D	L	F	y
1	1	1	−	−	−	−	y_{11}
2		2	−	−	−	+	y_{12}
3	2	1	+	−	−	−	y_{21}
4		2	+	−	−	+	y_{22}
5	3	1	−	+	−	−	y_{31}
6		2	−	+	−	+	y_{32}
7	4	1	+	+	−	−	y_{41}
8		2	+	+	−	+	y_{42}
9	5	1	−	−	+	−	y_{51}
10		2	−	−	+	+	y_{52}
11	6	1	+	−	+	−	y_{61}
12		2	+	−	+	+	y_{62}
13	7	1	−	+	+	−	y_{71}
14		2	−	+	+	+	y_{72}
15	8	1	+	+	+	−	y_{81}
16		2	+	+	+	+	y_{82}

R: ratio of microcrystalline cellulose to pregelatinized starch, MCC: PS
D: disintegrant type. PVPXL: crosslinked polyvinylpyrrolidone; CCS: croscarmellose sodium;
L: lubricant type. SSF: sodium stearyl fumarate; MS: magnesium stearate
F: dosage form: capsule or tablet
Y is %RS: percentage of related substances.

Chapter 6 showed that in two-level designs, the effect estimation could result from multiple pairs of one-factor-at-a-time experiments. Similarly, Table 7.2 indicates that the dosage form effect can be calculated as the average of the differences in the response within a whole plot. Across each whole plot where the other factors remained at the same level, the difference in the responses from two subplots should reflect the effect of using tablet over capsule as the dosage form, as in the case of the difference between y_{12} and y_{11}. A similar argument can be made for the lubricant effect, for example, by considering the difference between y_{51} and y_{11}. Note that all factors except the lubricant are at the same level for these two responses. There is, however, a disparity in these differences. Consider, for example, the first whole plot. If Yesim makes an error while setting the MCC:PS ratio, which is at the low level for that whole plot, and an 80:20 ratio was not achieved, her mistake will affect two experiments because we run two subplots within that whole plot.

Further, if this mistake in setting the correct ratio for example increases both responses by five, the responses for the two subplots corresponding to this whole plot will be $y_{12} + 5$ and $y_{11} + 5$. In calculating the effect of the dosage form, since we take the difference in the two responses, the increase in the responses will vanish and hence not contribute to the calculation of the dosage form effect. We can show that any error in a whole plot will get subtracted out when calculating the dosage form effect within a whole plot. We can further show that this will be the case for any effect calculated within a whole plot by taking the differences in the responses from subplots belonging to the same whole plot. However, we cannot say the same when calculating effects requiring pairwise differences from different whole plots. Consider, for example, the calculation of the lubricant effect in the case of the pair of responses, $y_{51,}$ and y_{11}. The error in setting the MCC:PS ratio in the first whole plot will only be present in y_{11} as we then have $y_{11} + 5$ as the response for the experiment. But since the same mistake does not affect y_{51}, as it does not come from the same whole plot, this error will remain intact in calculating the lubricant effect. This will be the case for any effect for which the analysis involves pairwise (one-factor-at-a-time) comparisons involving responses from different whole plots. Therefore, all effects should not be tested against the same error in a split-plot design. A more appropriate approach will be to separate the effects into two groups: effects that remain

Table 7.3: Separating the whole plot and subplot effects for the split-plot design in Table 7.1

Seven whole plot effects							Eight subplot effects							
RDL	DL	RL	RD	R	D	L	F	FR	FD	FL	FRD	FRL	FDL	FRDL
−	+	+	+	−	−	−	−	+	+	+	−	−	−	+
−	+	+	+	−	−	−	+	−	−	−	+	+	+	−
+	+	−	−	+	−	−	−	−	+	+	+	+	−	−
+	+	−	−	+	−	−	+	+	−	−	−	−	+	+
+	−	+	−	−	+	−	−	+	−	+	+	−	+	−
+	−	+	−	−	+	−	+	−	+	−	−	+	−	+
−	−	−	+	+	+	−	−	−	−	+	−	+	+	+
−	−	−	+	+	+	−	+	+	+	−	+	−	−	−
+	−	−	+	−	−	+	−	+	+	−	−	+	+	−
+	−	−	+	−	−	+	+	−	−	+	+	−	−	+
−	−	+	−	+	−	+	−	−	+	−	+	−	+	+
−	−	+	−	+	−	+	+	+	−	+	−	+	−	−
−	+	−	−	−	+	+	−	+	−	−	+	+	−	+
−	+	−	−	−	+	+	+	−	+	+	−	−	+	−
+	+	+	+	+	+	+	−	−	−	−	−	−	−	−
+	+	+	+	+	+	+	+	+	+	+	+	+	+	+

R: ratio of microcrystalline cellulose to pregelatinized starch, MCC: PS

D: disintegrant type. PVPXL: crosslinked polyvinylpyrrolidone; CCS: croscarmellose sodium;

L: lubricant type. SSF: sodium stearyl fumarate; MS: magnesium stearate

F: dosage form: capsule or tablet.

at the same level within a whole plot (whole-plot effects) and effects that change levels within a whole plot (subplot effects). In Table 7.3, we show all 15 effects in this design, and we can see that seven effects are whole-plot effects while the remaining eight effects are subplot effects. We then use two separate normal plots of the effects for these two groups, as shown in Figure 7.2.

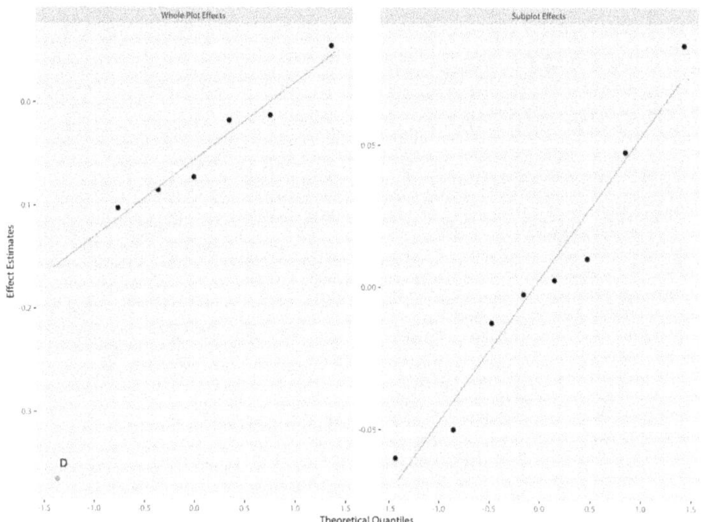

Figure 7.2: The normal plot of the whole-plot effects for percentage of related substances %RS shows disintegrant type. D seems to affect the %RS; the normal plot of the subplot effects for %RS shows the effects had no impact on %RS.

Look at the data

Rao urged Yesim to look at the data. As shown below, the data from Table 7.1 were reordered in descending order within each dosage form. The influence of the type of disintegrant is evident when comparing the D column to the dosage form columns F. Rao uses a dot plot to show the rationale for selecting CCS as the disintegrant with either the capsule or tablet dosage form.

D	F Capsule	F Tablet
	%RS	%RS
–	0.51	0.65
–	0.41	0.68
–	0.42	0.45
–	0.36	0.46
+	0.20	0.23
+	0.24	0.19
+	0.00	0.14
+	0.00	0.02
– (PVPXL)		
+ (CCS)		

CCS Capsule PVPXL Capsule

CCS Tablet PVPXL Tablet

0 0.17 0.34 0.51 0.68 %RS

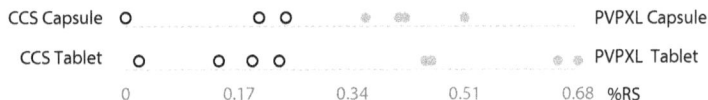

What to do next?

Yesim informed the project team that a capsule or tablet dosage form is viable, pending the final dose or strengths and feedback from the clinical and commercial departments. Yesim decided on the excipients for the formulation, including microcrystalline cellulose: pregelatinized starch 70:30, croscarmellose sodium, and magnesium stearate. Finally, once Yesim received the decision from the clinical and commercial departments, she started outlining plans for additional studies toward either dosage form.

Developing a Clinical Drug Product

Medbox Therapeutics acquired a molecule MBU2382 from Hill University. The Phase 1 clinical studies needed an immediate-release formulation.

The CMC team reviewed the physical and chemical characteristics of MBU238. They identified potential issues, including hydrolysis, the presence of secondary amines, oxidation, and pH-dependent solubility. They were aware of the possibility of accelerated development based on the Phase 2 results.

The CMC team outlined the following approach for developing the clinical product:

- Start the lab synthesis.
- Complete limited process work for the drug substance.
- Complete phase-appropriate analytical characterization of the drug substance.
- Initiate a drug excipient compatibility study.
- Based on the compatibility studies, plan studies to identify a clinical formulation.

Yesim was responsible for the last two activities.

Drug excipient compatibility study

Yesim decided to work toward a tablet formulation but also include excipients that could enable a capsule formulation. She went through the planning stages described in Chapter 6 and summarized some of the information outlined in Table 7.4 before meeting with Rao to discuss the project.

Table 7.4: Summary of factors, levels, and responses for an excipient compatibility study on MBU238

Drug Product	MBU238 clinical drug product		
Objective	Identify the excipients that are chemically compatible with MBU238.		
Factors	**Level (-)**	**Level (+)**	**Information**
Process	Wet granulation	Direct blend	
Diluent 1	Mannitol (M)	Pregelatinized starch (PS)	
Diluent 2	Microcrystalline cellulose (MCC)	Dicalcium phosphate (DP)	
Disintegrant	Cross-linked Polyvinylpyrrolidone (PVPXL)	Croscarmellose sodium (CCS)	
Lubricant	Stearic acid (SA)	Magnesium stearate (MS)	
Stabilizer	S1	S2	
Response Variable	**Measurement**	**Information**	**Initial criteria**
Percentage of related substances in 60 days	HPLC	Blends are stored in loosely capped glass vials at S1 (40°C/15%RH) and S2 (40°C/75%RH) for 30 days.	Minimize related substances
Experimental Design	**Trials**	**Data Analysis**	**Interpretation**
Seven factors, two-level	Can do 20 trials	Tables, graphs, statistical analysis	Statistical and subject matter

The experimental design, setup, and data

Yesim approached Rao to discuss how to design the experiment. The experimental setup would involve seven factors. If Yesim tested all seven factors at two levels, a complete factorial design would require $2^7 = 128$ trials, which is excessive. Rao realized that the first six factors are related to the formulation of the blend, whereas the last factor, storage condition (40°C/15%RH vs. 40°C/75%RH), can be applied once a blend is prepared and split into two. This suggests that they run these experiments using a split-plot design where storage condition is a subplot factor. This may indeed provide some relief in experimental efforts; however, even in this scenario, they will still need to have $2^6 = 64$ whole plots to run.

Recall the half fraction designs we covered in Chapter 6. The number of trials can be cut in half by sacrificing an effect (i.e., not estimating the effect) and creating some confounding, among other effects. A half fraction would, in this case, require 32 experiments. Yesim deemed this number also excessive. Rao then suggested a 2^{6-2}, a quarter fraction design outlined in Table 7.5. Note that the reduction in the number of experiments goes in the power of two: a half fraction, quarter fraction, and so forth. The main reason for this is the way we obtained these fractions. In designing the half fraction, we considered an effect that would be sacrificed and often picked the highest order interaction deemed least likely to be significant. Since in two-level designs, all effects are tested at an equal number of low and high levels, we could pick any effect and choose half of the experiments for which this effect was always at either the high or low level, hence "sacrificing" the effect, as we cannot estimate the impact of an effect on the response if it does not change at all. If we followed the same strategy, we could use one effect to obtain the half fraction in which all other effects

Table 7.5: A $2^{6-2} \times 2^1$ split-plot design to evaluate the effect of the process, diluent ratios, disintegrant, lubricant, and stabilizer type on MBU238 mixtures stored at 40°C/15%RH and 40°C/75%RH for 60 days. %RS is percentage of related substance

Trial	Order	Process	Diluents 1	Diluents 2	Disintegrant	Lubricant	Stabilizer	40°C/15%RH		40°C/75%RH	
		E=ABC	D	F=BCD	B	C	A	%RS1	%RS2	%RS1	%RS2
1	8	−	−	−	−	−	−	0.07	0.03	2.42	0.03
2	6	+	−	−	−	−	+	0.85	0.42	3.00	0.31
3	1	+	−	+	+	−	−	0.05	0.03	0.84	0.15
4	12	−	−	+	+	−	+	1.27	0.18	3.14	0.17
5	11	+	−	+	−	+	−	0.01	0.03	1.10	0.05
6	13	−	−	+	−	+	+	0.07	0.08	6.14	0.26
7	9	−	−	−	+	+	−	0.01	0.03	3.04	0.19
8	4	+	−	−	+	+	+	0.21	0.22	1.52	0.56
9	14	−	+	+	−	−	−	0.04	0.03	2.22	0.16
10	3	+	+	+	−	−	+	0.75	0.15	3.92	0.51
11	7	+	+	−	+	−	−	0.15	0.03	1.08	0.05
12	10	−	+	−	+	−	+	1.53	0.17	3.86	0.35
13	15	+	+	−	−	+	−	0.01	0.03	0.84	0.11
14	16	−	+	−	−	+	+	0.18	0.31	4.98	0.36
15	2	−	+	+	+	+	−	0.01	0.03	3.34	0.24
16	5	+	+	+	+	+	+	0.30	0.09	3.20	0.11

would be tested at two levels an equal number of times. We would then use one of these effects to halve the half fraction further and obtain the quarter fraction. Similarly, we would get one eighth, one/16th, and so forth fractions of a two-level full factorial design. In the half fraction, sacrificing an effect also led to confounding among other effects; since we sacrificed two effects in obtaining a quarter fraction, confounding relationships can get complicated, particularly for high-order fractionation. We, therefore, recommend product developers seeking to generate quarter or higher-order fractions consult a book or software.

A blend was prepared for every trial and stored in containers in two stability chambers maintained at 40°C/15%RH and 40°C/75%RH, respectively. Samples from the stability chambers were pulled at periodic intervals. Table 7.5 shows the data for samples stored and analyzed after 30 days. The samples were analyzed using a chromatographic method. The information for two related substances was computed from the chromatograms and reported as %RS1 and %RS2. Given the change in %RS1 on stability between the experiments, Yesim suggested Rao focus on analyzing %RS1.

Analysis

As explained in Figure 7.2, two separate normal plots are needed because the effects are classified into two categories. Figure 7.3 shows the normal plot of the whole-plot effects and the subplot effects separately.

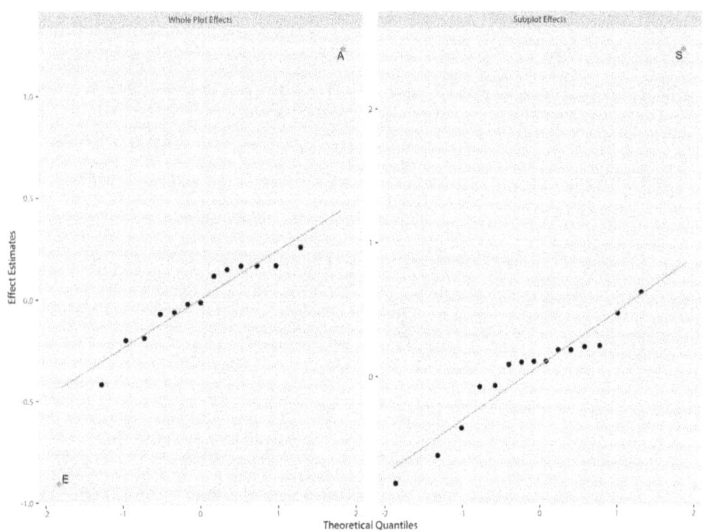

Figure 7.3: The normal plot of the whole-plot effects for %RS1 shows Stabilizer A and Process E seem to affect %RS1; the normal plot of the subplot effects for %RS1 shows storage condition S seems to affect %RS1.

Look at the data

Based on the normal plots in Figure 7.3, Rao rearranged Table 7.5 as a replicated $2^2 \times 2^1$ split-plot design with the data in descending order across the rows within each storage condition for MBU238 blends. Rao and Yesim reviewed the rearranged table and the corresponding trellis plot in Figure 7.4, focusing on %RS1. Rao used the cross in each panel of the trellis plot in Figure 7.4 to indicate the average response of the whole-plot effects at its low and high levels. This helped Yesim observe the potential significance of the main effect and the deviation from the average in the response for each experiment.

Process	Stabilizer	%RS1 at 40°C/15%RH				%RS1 at 40°C/75%RH			
–	–	0.07	0.04	0.01	0.01	3.34	3.04	2.42	2.22
+	–	0.15	0.05	0.01	0.01	1.10	1.08	0.84	0.84
–	+	1.53	1.27	0.18	0.07	6.14	4.98	3.86	3.14
+	+	0.85	0.75	0.30	0.21	3.92	3.20	3.00	1.52
– (Wet)	– (S1)								
+ (Dry)	+ (S2)								

The analysis revealed the following. First, Stabilizer 1 seemed to be more effective than Stabilizer 2 in protecting the molecule from a chemical reaction. Additionally, Stabilizer 2 showed more variability than Stabilizer 1, indicating a need for a higher concentration for Stabilizer 2. The higher %RS1 in the wet granulation and 40°C/75%RH samples compared to the dry blend and 40°C/15%RH samples indicated the molecule might be susceptible to hydrolysis.

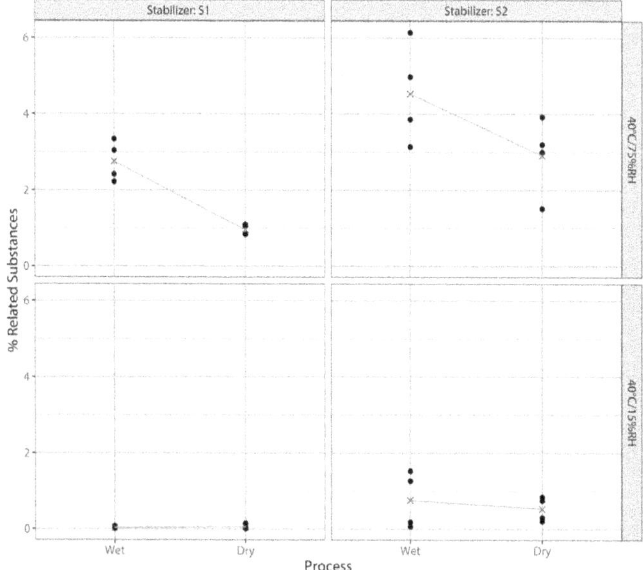

Figure 7.4: The trellis plot shows the effect of the two stabilizers on the percentage of related substances for two different storage conditions.

What to do next

The data analysis helped Yesim decide on the process and the formulation composition for MBU238 tablets. She decided to do the following:

- Develop a dry blend process.
- Use a combination of microcrystalline cellulose and pregelatinized starch as the diluent with Stabilizer 1.
- Use croscarmellose sodium as the disintegrant. This is to prevent an oxidation reaction during product storage, which could occur if future lots of cross-linked polyvinylpyrrolidone could have residual peroxide.
- Use magnesium stearate as the lubricant.
- Evaluate the need to include a desiccant when packaging the product in high-density polyethylene HDPE bottles.
- Manufacture 3 kg of uncoated tablets and evaluate the photostability of the product with and without coating components.
- Complete a study to determine the effects of varying the percentage of the formulation components.

Evaluating the photostability of the product

Yesim and Cliff, the operator, manufactured 3 kg of uncoated tablets. The yield was 2.7 kg; this was separated into two 1.35 kg batches. They completed a coating trial with each batch, Trials 1 and 2, outlined in Table 7.6. Samples from each trial were subjected to a photostability test with the corresponding controls. The control tablets were wrapped in aluminum foil. The data showed that it is necessary to coat the tablets with a coating suspension containing iron oxide pigment.

Table 7.6: Evaluating the effect of the coating formulation on the photostability of MBU238 tablets

Trial	Coating suspension	Pigment	Comment	%RS1 Control	%RS1 after 10h Xenon
Control	None	None	Uncoated tablet	0.40	9.65
1	Coating suspension with an opacifier	None	Coated tablet	0.38	1.76
2	Coating suspension with an opacifier	Yellow iron oxide	Coated tablet	0.32	0.47

Evaluating the formulation robustness

Once the formulation composition was identified, Yesim needed to confirm that no stability issues arose within a specific quantitative range of each excipient. This would ensure the formulation's robustness. As shown in Table 7.7, Yesim and Cliff completed a 2^3 factorial design with stability and dissolution as the two responses.

Experimental Data

Table 7.7: A 2^3 factorial design to confirm the robustness of the MBU238 tablet formulation

Trial	Order	R	D	L	% dissolved at 20 min		%RS1	
		Ratio	%	%	Initial	3 months	Initial	3 months
1	5	–	–	–	73	71	0.37	0.32
2	4	+	–	–	69	74	0.45	0.34
3	3	–	+	–	74	75	0.41	0.36
4	6	+	+	–	75	69	0.33	0.38
5	8	–	–	+	71	74	0.41	0.40
6	2	+	–	+	72	73	0.33	0.45
7	1	–	+	+	70	71	0.29	0.41
8	7	+	+	+	73	75	0.39	0.36
	–	70:30	3.5	0.75				
	+	50:50	5.0	1.25				

Analysis

For the analysis of both percentage dissolved at 20 min and percentage of RS1, Rao used the difference in the measurement at three months and the initial measurement. The normal plots of the effects for the two responses are given in Figure 7.5. In both cases they indicate no significant effect and confirm the tablet formulation's robustness relative to the factors considered in the experiments, and it is concluded that no formulation refinement is needed.

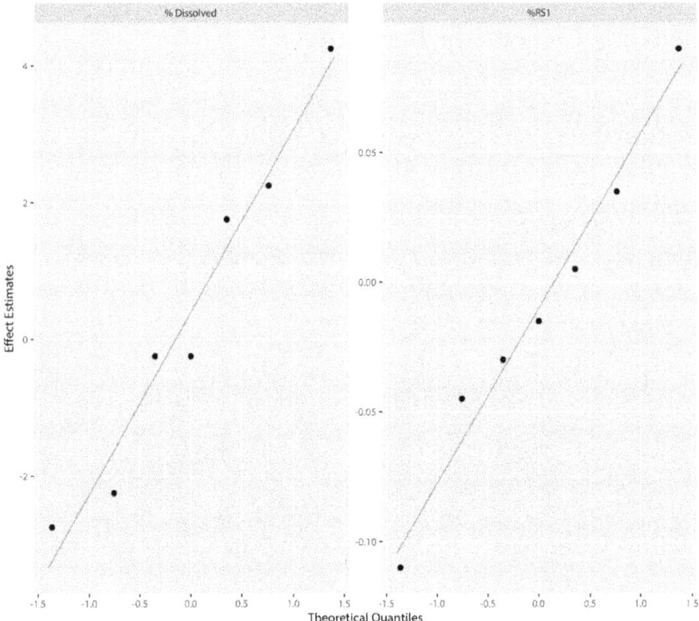

Figure 7.5: The normal plots of the effects for percentage dissolved at 20 min and percentage of RS1 show no factors affected the percentage dissolved at 20 min and percentage of RS1, confirming the robustness of the BU238 tablet formulation.

An Introduction to Blocking

During the early stages of development, the chemist at Medbox Therapeutics synthesized two lots of the compound XCD2356-8. They sent both lots over to Yesim so that she could explore initial formulations, indicating that the two lots of the compound could have different amounts of total process impurities. Once Yesim decided the number of excipients to test, she realized there was enough to do four trials using the first lot and five trials using the second lot. But each lot had different amounts of process-related impurities. Yesim approached Rao with the question of how to accommodate these two lots in an eight-run trial knowing the raw material had different amounts of total process impurities, and which might affect the product stability.

Rao explained blocking to Yesim, a process that would eliminate the effect of inhomogeneities in the experimental material. In this case, Yesim executed four trials with one lot of drug substance and the remaining four trials with a second lot of drug substance. The objective of blocking is to account for the effects of nuisance factors that in this case characterize the experimental material. The group of homogenous material (drug substance lot in this case) is called a block. In this example, a two-factor interaction (DB) between the diluent and binder would be confounded with the difference between the two blocks. Rao described blocking as a filter to eliminate unwanted disturbances, reducing the influence of variability coming from the experimental material, environment, or process. Rao indicated blocking arrangements were available for all 2^k ($k>1$) factorial designs.

Yesim prepared and stored the eight blends as outlined in Table 7.8. The response was percentage related substances %RS.

Experimental Data

Table 7.8: A 2^{4-1} design to identify the excipients for a formulation blocked on two lots of drug substance

Block = DB (DS lots)	Trial	Order	D	B	L	T (DBL)	%RS
1	2	4	+	−	−	+	1.310
1	3	1	−	+	−	+	0.977
1	6	3	+	−	+	−	1.002
1	7	2	−	+	+	−	1.160
2	1	1	−	−	−	−	0.167
2	4	3	+	+	−	−	2.248
2	5	2	−	−	+	+	0.119
2	8	4	+	+	+	+	2.143
		−	M/S	HPC	SA	SSG	
		+	D/S	PVP	MS	CCS	

DS: drug substance; D: diluent; B: binder; L: lubricant; T: disintegrant
M/S: microcrystalline cellulose/pregelatinized starch (65:35);
D/S: dicalcium phosphate/pregelatinized starch (80:20)
HPC: hydroxypropyl cellulose; PVP: polyvinylpyrrolidone
SA: stearic acid; MS: magnesium stearate
SSG: sodium starch glycolate; CCS: croscarmellose sodium
%RS: percentage of related substances after 8 weeks at 40°C/75%RH

Analysis

Once the analytical chemist provided the data from the stability studies, Rao employed the normal plot of the effects to analyze the data, as shown in Figure 7.6. We can see that the diluent and the binder may have an effect on %RS present after eight weeks (see "If you wondered," p. 115, for additional discussion on blocking and confounding as well as the statistical analysis.)

Look at the data

Yesim and Rao projected the 2^{4-1} factorial design in Table 7.8 to a replicated 2^2 factorial design because only the binder and disintegrant were significant. They drew a cube plot

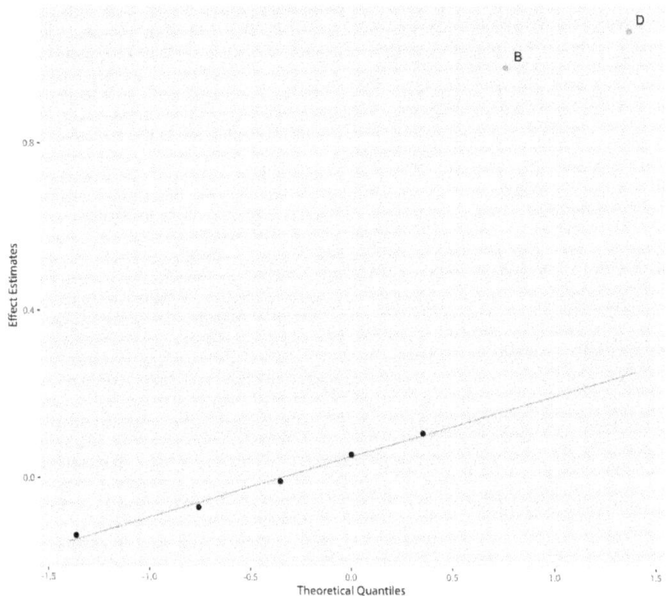

Figure 7.6: The normal plot of the effects for the percentage of related substance %RS shows the diluent and binder seem to affect the %RS for a formulation blocked on two lots of drug substance.

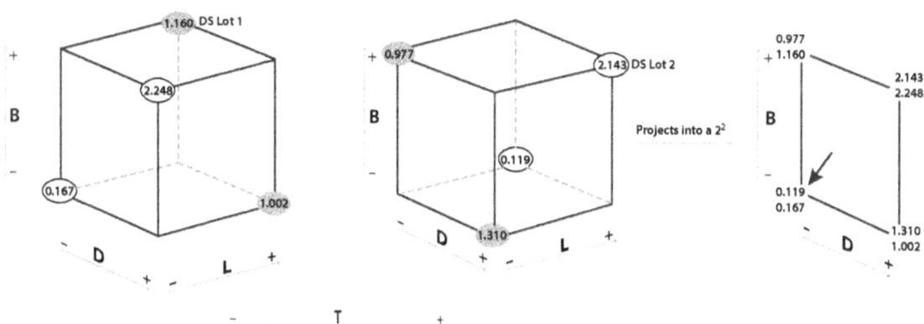

Figure 7.7: The 2^{4-1} factorial design projected to a replicated 2^2 design. The arrow indicates the lowest %RS.

projected to a square plot to visualize the effect of the two factors on percentage of related substances (Figure 7.7.) The lowest percentage of related substances was observed when using microcrystalline cellulose and pregelatinized start with hydroxypropyl cellulose (indicated by the arrow on the left of the square). The use of dicalcium phosphate (a basic excipient) or polyvinylpyrrolidone increased the percentage of related substances on storage. These conclusions are based on visual tools. They are usually supported by a rigorous statistical analysis and experimental confirmation.

What to do next

Based on the data and analysis, Yesim decided to include microcrystalline cellulose, pregelatinized starch, hydroxypropyl cellulose, sodium starch glycolate, and magnesium stearate in the next series of experiments to develop the drug product. The team tentatively concluded that the block effect was not significant, as the average responses for the two blocks were not too different, acknowledging that rigorous statistical analysis might show otherwise, and assumed that the process impurities in the drug substance did not become impurities or degradants in the formulation. Blocking provided a broader basis for their inference.

Had there been a significant block effect, implications would have been minimal, since the variation between blocks is a nuisance factor, that is, a factor we are not necessarily interested in. First, the result would have confirmed our initial speculation on the impact on the variation in composition in the lots. Hence, the conclusions we obtained from our analysis can be considered more reliable than in the case of completely randomized designs where the known differences in the lot are not accounted for. Secondly, the result would have indicated how Yesim should run experiments in the future if different lots are involved. Finally, even though the block effect is considered a nuisance factor, the group would work toward reducing and stabilizing the percentage of process impurities in each drug substance lot.

If you wondered

Constructing a normal plot (Figure 7.6) in Microsoft® Excel®

Step	Column	Description
1	A	Arrange the effects in ascending order
2	B	Type in the position (i) of the ordered effects
3	C	Calculate the cumulative probability f_i = (i-0.375)/(n+0.25)
4	D	Use the NORM.S.INV(f_i) function to find the z-score
5	Plot	Plot the ordered effects on the vertical axis and the corresponding z-score on the horizontal axis

A		B	C	D
Effects		Position	f_i	z-score
DL	−0.1370	1	0.09	−1.36
L	−0.0695	2	0.22	−0.76
T	−0.0070	3	0.36	−0.35
DB (block)	0.0570	4	0.50	0.00
DT	0.1085	5	0.64	0.35
B	0.9825	6	0.78	0.76
D	1.0700	7	0.91	1.36

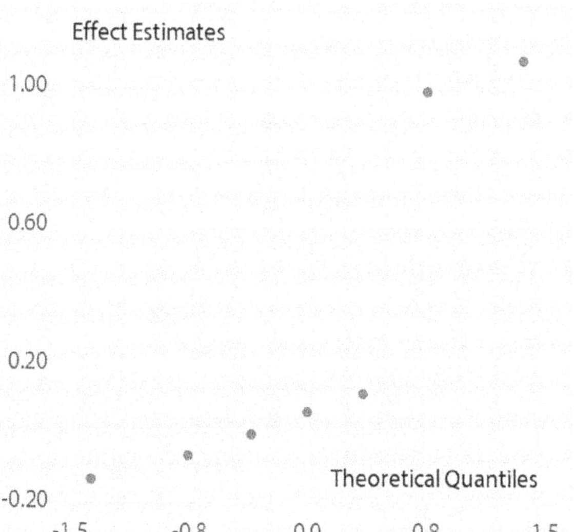

More on Blocking

The normal plot in Figure 7.6 only considers seven effects. A two-level design with four factors would have 15 effects: four main effects, 6 two-factor interactions, 4 three-factor interactions, and 1 four-factor interaction. The table below shows the design matrix from Table 7.8, including all effects with interaction effects obtained by entry-wise multiplication of the corresponding main effect columns.

D	B	L	T	DB	DL	DT	BL	BT	LT	DBL	DBT	DLT	BLT	DBLT
+	−	−	+	−	−	+	+	−	−	+	−	−	+	+
−	+	−	+	−	+	−	−	+	−	+	−	+	−	+
+	−	+	−	−	+	−	−	+	−	−	+	−	+	+
−	+	+	−	−	−	+	+	−	−	−	+	+		+
−	−	−	−	+	+	+	+	+	+	−	−	−	+	+
+	+	−	−	+	−	−	−	−	+	−	−	+	−	+
−	−	+	+	+	−	−	−	−	+	+	+	−	+	+
+	+	+	+	+	+	+	+	+	+	+	+	+	−	+

This table indicates that the DBLT effect did not change levels throughout the design and hence is not estimable. This is by design, as we picked this highest order interaction as the generator to obtain the half fraction of the 2^4 full factorial design. As a result, we also noticed that the effects are "paired." The column representing the main effect of D is the same as the column representing the BLT interaction. Hence, these two effects are confounded. Similarly, there are seven pairs of effects sharing the same column. This was expected based on Yesim and Rao's decision to use only eight rather than 16 experiments. With fewer experiments, the number of effects that can be estimated will also be fewer, as fewer experiments provide less information than twice as many experiments. The eight experiments allow for only the estimation of seven pairs of effects and not the individual effects; this is a reasonable trade-off given the cost of more experiments. Nevertheless, lowering the number of experiments from 16 to eight made it impossible to estimate all effects.

We also added one more feature to the design: We ran the experiments in two blocks rather than in a completely randomized way as would have been conventionally required. This was to avoid the impact of the variation on the batch of raw material. Hence, we aimed to gain more accuracy in our estimation of the effects by controlling the levels of the nuisance factor (variation in the batch of raw material) and running specific experiments at each level. We expect this offered a fairer comparison of the effects of interest within those levels. However, we can see that the BD interaction does not change levels within the blocks. This was once again by design, as we picked this effect to obtain the two blocks; whenever the BD effect was at the low level, we ran those four experiments using one batch of raw material, and whenever it was at the high level, we used the other batch. We deliberately confounded the potential block effect (high variation due to batch-to-batch variation) with the BD effect. Another effect, LT, was also confounded with the block effect because it remained at a specific level within the blocks. That was also expected, as in the half fraction design, BD and LT were confounded. LT is confounded with the block effect, and so is BD. Coming back to the seven effects in the normal probability plot, those correspond to the seven pairs of confounded effect. Hence, a more accurate depiction of significant effects would be D + BLT and B + DLT. However, if we assume that the three-factor interactions are not likely to be significant, we can attribute all the significance to the main effects of D and B, as we did. Moreover, one of the seven pairs on the normal probability plot is the BD + LT pair or, more accurately, Block Effect + BD + LT.

Now that we have identified B and D as potentially significant effects, we can use the analysis of variance to test for their statistical significance. The ANOVA for the model with B and D only is given below. Low *p*-values confirm the significance of these effects. Please note that *p*-values do not measure the size of an effect or the importance of the result. We provide the residual analysis for this example on the book's website datatodecision.org, to confirm the model assumptions imposed on the experimental error.

	Sum of squares	Degrees of freedom	Mean squares	F-ratio	*p*-value
D	2.29	1	2.29	114.5	~10^{-4}
B	1.93	1	1.93	96.5	~10^{-4}
Error	0.08	5	0.02		
Total	4.30	7			

NOTES

Allen, L.V. and Ansel, H.C., (2013). *Ansel's Pharmaceutical Dosage Forms and Drug Delivery Systems.* Tenth edition. New York: Wolters Kluwer Health.

Augsburger, L. L., Hoag, S. W. ed. (2008). *Pharmaceutical Dosage Forms: Tablets, Volume 2.* Third edition. Florida: CRC Press.

Byrn, S. R., Zografi, G., and Chen, X. (2017). *Solid-State Properties of Pharmaceuticals.* New Jersey: Wiley.

Cleveland, W.S. (1993). *Visualizing Data*. New Jersey: Hobart Press.

Kulahci, M. and Menon, A. (2017). Trellis plots as visual aids for analyzing split-plot experiments. *Quality Engineering* 29(2): 211-225.

Montgomery, D. (2009). *Design and Analysis of Experiments*. New York: Wiley.

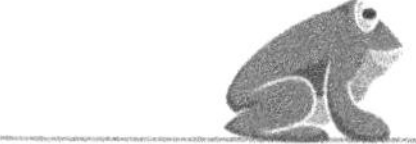

Reasonable, if not rational, decisions are taken during development.

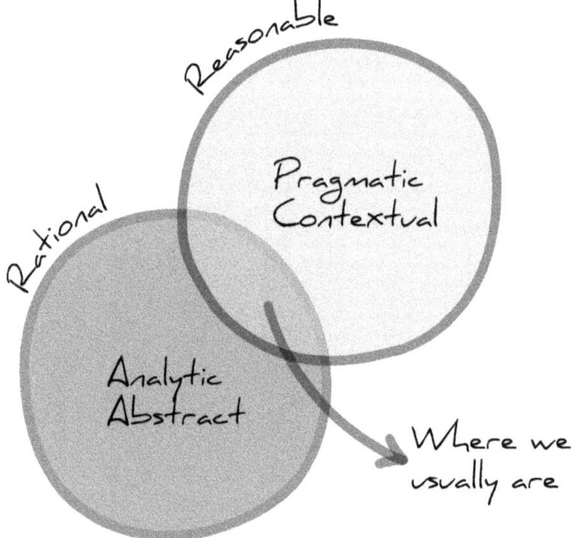

8

How Does Experimental Design Enable Process Development?

Early process development studies help gather empirical data and knowledge generalized across various conditions during process characterization and scale-up. Process development occurs in stages across the product development cycle, as outlined in Chapter 3 and below.

Early process development	Identify a process and the initial operating ranges.
Process characterization studies	Characterize the process, and complete initial scale-up trials.
Process robustness studies	Complete scale-up studies toward commercial manufacturing.
Registration stability batches	Long-term stability studies for the to-be-marketed product.
Commercial scale-up	Scale-up at the industrial site.
Validation batches	Verify a reproducible commercial manufacturing process.

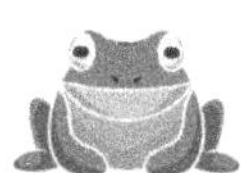

Process development may not follow the above stages sequentially. For example, the characterization and robustness studies can be combined, as can the commercial scale-up and validation batches. Scale-up from the laboratory to pilot to commercial scale depends on the subject matter knowledge of the chemist, formulator, operators, and engineers. Experimental designs provide a structure for gathering evidence at the various stages of process development, as outlined in Table 8.1. The structured approach enables CMC drug product regulatory submissions and successful commercial manufacture.

Table 8.1 shows us that experimental design is extensively used in process development and troubleshooting. Experimental design offers a solid yet flexible framework that guides the route toward process understanding enabling product development and manufacturing.

Pharmaceutical processes consist of a sequence of steps. The output from one processing step is the input for the next processing step. For example, a three-step process would be granulation, compression, and coating. Additional manufacturing steps include putting the coated tablets into bottles, labeling, secondary packaging, and distribution. Judgments are made in designing the experimental trials based on technical knowledge, available resources, batch size, yield, testing, and amount of material used in each processing step.

Process development for an immediate release tablet

Yesim had to develop a fluid-bed wet granulation process for one of Medbox's therapeutics products. She was aware that trials might not go as planned, and that circumstances involving facility, equipment, raw materials, or operators might result in flawed trials. Rao counseled her to block when in doubt, because

Table 8.1: An outline for the process development studies from formulation development to validation batches

	Product/ formulation development	Early process development	Process characterization studies	Initial scale-up*	Process robustness studies*	Commercial transfer and scale-up	Validation batches
Objective	Develop the product/ formulation.	Identify a process for clinical supplies.	Evaluate the effect of process and formulation parameters on the quality measures.	Scale-up	Evaluate process and formulation robustness on quality measures.	Industrial scale-up to support operating ranges for commercial manufacture.	Confirm process parameters for commercial manufacturing.
Approximate Scale**	Laboratory 5 to 100 g	Laboratory 20 to 1000 g	Laboratory and Pilot Plant 50 g to 2 kg	Pilot Plant 2 to 10 kg	Laboratory and Pilot Plant 2 to 20 kg	Industrial Site	Industrial Site
An estimate for the number of Trials*	12 to 24	2 to 6	8 to 24	2 to 12	8 to 24	2 to 6	≥3. Decided based on process development
Design(s)	Fractional Factorials, One-at-a-time plans, Optimal, Split-Plot, Definitive Screening Designs						
Analysis Tools	Technical knowledge, numerical and graphical summaries						
Factors	Selected based on excipients and process.	Selected based on process parameters.	Selected based on process parameters and excipients.	Selected based on process parameters.	Selected based on process parameters, drug substance, and excipients.	Selected based on process parameters.	Not applicable.
Quality measures	Physical characterization, dosage form performance, stability markers, and Certificate of Analysis testing (when applicable).						

*Registration stability batches are usually manufactured during this period.

**These are guidelines because the design that fits the objective and resources decides the batch size and the number of trials arranging the trials in blocks is a practical risk management tool.

During process development trials where a significant amount of drug substance and other resources are consumed, blocking is a risk management policy to limit the consequence of mistakes or interrupted trials because of equipment failures, budget changes, or revised goals:

1. If something goes wrong with one or more trials within a block, only the affected block must be repeated.
2. Arrange the trials so that if the trials end prematurely, the experimenter still has useful blocks to analyze. The partially completed design should have a high salvage content.

Experimental Data

Yesim identified five factors for the first fluid-bed trial at a 2 kg batch size and had sufficient resources to complete 16 trials. The scheduling of the trials allowed the team to complete four trials in one week. Rao suggested arranging the trials in four blocks and arranging the first two blocks as an eight-trial 2^{5-2} in keeping with his recommendation of a partially completed design with high salvage content. Table 8.2 shows the design and the responses. The assumption here is that blocks do not interact with factors. Blocks 3 and 4 of Table 8.2 represent planned but not executed trials.

After completing the first eight trials, Yesim found that the fluid bed could not maintain the inlet temperature during the trial. Upon inspection, Lina from the maintenance department found the issue and estimated that parts and repairs would take 5 days. This would delay the trials by more than 2 weeks because other projects were in the queue as well. Since no alternative equipment was available and the trials were designed in blocks,

Yesim and Rao decided to analyze the first eight trials and determine if there was enough information to decide whether to conduct the scale-up trials planned for the next stage of development. The target d_{50} particle size was 150 to 250 microns, and percentage dissolved at 30 min Q30 was 65%.

Table 8.2: A 2^{5-1} design in four blocks to evaluate the effect of fluid-bed process parameters on the granule particle size and dissolution. The first two blocks constitute a quarter fraction, 2^{5-2}

Block = MA (Weeks)	Trial	Order	P	M	A	S (PM)	T (PA)	PS μ	Q30 %
1	3	3	−	+	−	−	+	103	80
1	4	1	+	+	−	+	−	321	65
1	5	4	−	−	+	+	−	50	79
1	6	2	+	−	+	−	+	217	72
2	1	7	−	−	−	+	+	84	81
2	2	5	+	−	−	−	−	245	70
2	7	6	−	+	+	−	−	141	78
2	8	8	+	+	+	+	+	294	69
3	9	9	−	−	−	+	−		
3	10	10	+	−	−	+	+		
3	15	11	−	+	+	+	−		
3	16	12	+	+	+	+	+		
4	11	13	−	+	−	+	+		
4	12	16	+	+	−	+	−		
4	13	15	−	−	+	+	+		
4	14	14	+	−	+	+	−		
		−	3	5	1	20	45		
		+	6	2	3	60	60		

P: percentage of binder
M: percentage of final moisture
A: atomization pressure, psi
S: spray rate g/min
T: inlet temperature °C
PS: average particle size d_{50} calculated from log probability plots
Q30: percentage dissolved at 30 min

Analysis and Interpretation

The normal plot in Figure 8.1 indicates that the percentages of binder and final moisture seem to affect the granule particle size. An increase in the percentage of binder increases the cohesion between particles, enhances powder agglomeration, and increases the granule size. On average, an increase in the final moisture content results in larger granules because of the lower drying time and less granule attrition in the fluid-bed chamber. The increased percentage of binder reduces the dissolution rate on average (Figure 8.1). However, all Q30 values in Table 8.2 met the 65% target.

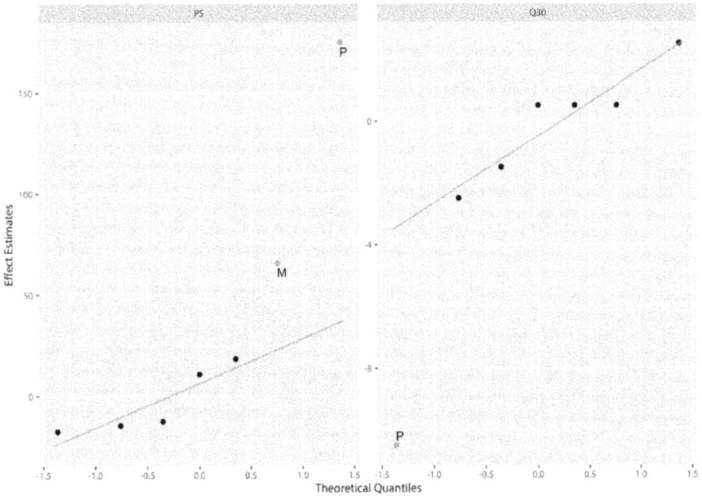

Figure 8.1: The normal plot of the effects for particle size PS shows the percentage of binder P and percentage of final moisture M seem to affect the d_{50} PS, and the normal plot of the effects for percentage dissolved at 30 min Q30 shows the percentage of binder P seems to affect Q30.

What to do next

Yesim decided to use a 5% binder and a higher percentage of final moisture and evaluate the inlet temperature, atomization pressure, and spray rate for the scale-up trials.

Initial Scale-up and Process Robustness

The batch size for the initial scale-up study for the fluid-bed process scale-up study was 25 kg. Yesim wanted to study three factors: the inlet temperature, T, the atomization pressure, A, and the spray rate, S. Based on the dose, there was enough drug substance to conduct six trials. Rao suggested a $3(2^{3-2})$ design, that is, Rao reminded Yesim of the geometric figure in Chapter 6 (obtuse wedge as a bisected regular tetrahedron, p. 79). These designs are called John's three-quarter fractional factorials. Rao's proposed design can estimate the three main effects clear of each other and of two-factor interactions, but the two-factor interactions are confounded. The estimated effects are T, A, S (confounded with TAS), TA, and TS (confounded with AS). The three-factor interaction (TAS) is assumed to be negligible.

Experimental Data

Table 8.2 shows John's three-quarter fractional factorial and the responses. The Q30 values for the six trials ranged from 68% to 76%, and the assay values ranged from 95.4% to 102%.

Table 8.2: A $3(2^{3-2})$ fractional factorial to evaluate a fluid-bed process

Trial	Order	T	A	S	PS, μ	A geometric view
1	2	–	–	–	239	
2	6	+	–	–	193	
3	3	–	+	–	132	
6	4	+	–	+	212	
7	1	–	+	+	145	
8	5	+	+	+	187	
	–	50	2.5	110		
	+	60	3.5	160		

T: inlet temperature, °C
A: atomization pressure, bar
S: spray rate, g/min
PS, μ: particle size in microns

Analysis and Interpretation

We have mostly considered two-level factorial designs, where the number of experiments is always a power of two. John's three-quarter replicates offer additional options when the number of experiments that can be run cannot be a power of two. Using three of the four quarters of a given full or fractional factorial design leads to a saving of experimental trials equivalent to the quarter fraction of the base design. If conducted with some care, these quarter replicates can offer estimates of the main effects and two-factor interactions, assuming interactions between three or more factors are negligible. The estimation of these effects would require the use of some but not necessarily all of these replicates. For example, using Trials 1, 2, 7, and 8, the main effect of T can be estimated free from confounding with other main effects and two-factor interactions. Nonetheless, testing for the statistical significance of the effects will be very challenging in this particular design, given there are only six experiments. Therefore, we will limit the analysis to a visual evaluation of the experimental results combined with the target d_{50} particle size.

Yesim was interested in finding the factor settings to obtain a d_{50} target particle size of 150 to 250 microns and decided to look at the data. She studied the cube plot in Figure 8.2 and reasoned that having a high atomization pressure results in small droplet sizes of the binder, which reduces the number of particles that can be agglomerated and could result in a smaller granule particle size (132μ and 145μ).

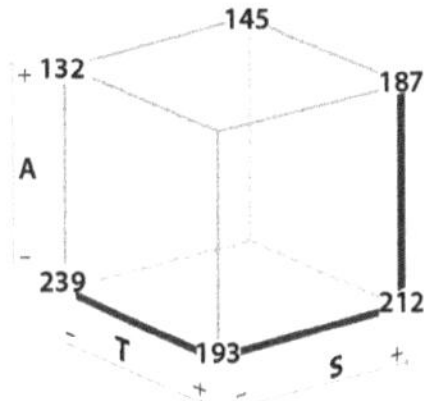

Figure 8.2: Cube plot of the $3(2^{3-2})$ fractional factorial evaluating a fluid-bed scale-up process. The highlighted edges indicate operating at a higher temperature T+, A–, and S– to obtain the target d_{50} particle size range of 150 to 200 microns.

Given the smaller d_{50} particle size at T-, A- (239μ) compared to T–, A+ (132μ,145μ) and the relatively similar particle size at T+, A– (193μ, 212μ) and T+, A + (187μ), she studied the TA interaction plot (Figure 8.3). Assuming a potential interaction between atomization A and temperature T, she reasoned that at higher temperatures, the evaporation rate of the binder solution would cancel the influence of the atomization pressure on the d_{50} granule particle size. She hypothesized a high inlet temperature would reduce the impact of the atomization pressure on the d_{50} particle size. She decided on operating at T+, A–, and S– (Trial 2) pending confirmation during the scale-up trials to 110 kg.

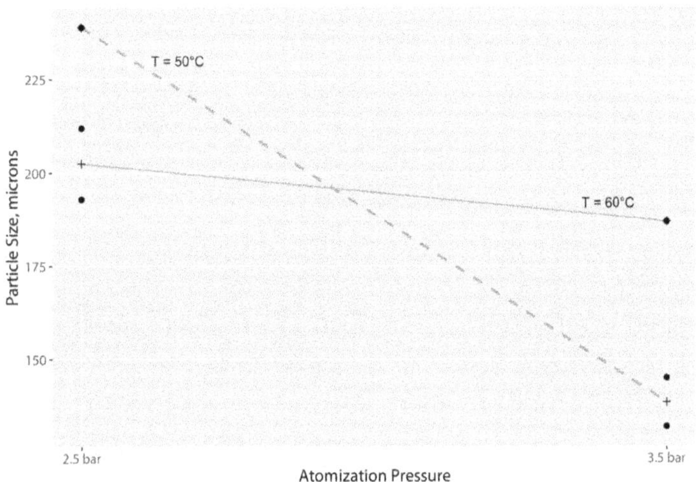

Figure 8.3: The plot indicates a potential interaction between atomization A and temperature T. "•" represents the six experimental data points, and "+" represents the average when applicable.

What to do next

The particle size distribution, bulk and tap density, and porosity measurements for Trials 2 (d_{50} = 193 microns), 6 (d_{50} = 212 microns), and 8 (d_{50} = 187 microns) were similar. The product from Trials 2, 6, and 8 were combined and used for the subsequent process development trials. Each of the 25 kg trials had an 85% yield approximately. Combining the three trials gave Yesim 64 kg of the blend for compression trials.

Scale-up for compression

While manufacturing Phase 3 supplies, Yesim noticed that the acceptable quality level (AQL) on the appearance of compressed uncoated tablets was higher than in previous campaigns. The batches passed AQL testing, but she anticipated issues during commercial manufacture. Changing the formulation composition or exploring the drug substance morphology and particle size was not an option at this stage of product development. She decided to compare the effectiveness of a treatment applied to the tooling for eliminating or reducing the major defects observed with untreated tooling. The team decided to conduct compression trials using a tablet press with ≥ 50,000 tablets/hour output. Tablet appearance was assessed by AQL testing (see "If you wondered," p. 138, for a partial list of visual defects.)

Experimental Data

Table 8.3 shows the percentage of major defects from the AQL testing. Other tablet characteristics were within the acceptance criteria, including weight, hardness, friability, assay, related substances, and uniformity of dosage units.

Table 8.3: Percentage of defects (major and critical) from AQL testing on uncoated tablets compressed with untreated (UT) and treated (T) tooling. This is a split-split plot design of $2^1 \times 2^1 \times 2^1$

Trial	Tooling	Compression Speed			
		−		+	
		Hardness		Hardness	
		−	+	−	+
1	UT	0.40	0.35	0.75	0.60
2	T	0.00	0.00	0.00	0.01

H: hardness, kP
T: type of tooling, untreated UT vs. treated T

Analysis

Due to the limited number of experiments and no replications, it is difficult to conduct a rigorous statistical analysis of the experimental data. However, considering the small variation in the data in Table 8.3, Yesim concluded that the tooling treatment eliminated the uncoated tablets' defects at different compression speeds and hardness levels.

What to do next?

Treated tooling sets were used for additional studies and the proposed commercial manufacture. Further studies evaluating pre-compression force and the speed of the force feeder were completed to justify the normal operating and proven acceptable ranges.

The uncoated tablets from Trial 2 in Table 8.3 were combined for the coating studies to justify the proven acceptable ranges of the coating parameters.

Scale-up for coating

Yesim had to complete film-coating trials with the uncoated tablets from Trials 3 and 4 (Table 8.3) to establish the proven acceptable ranges (PAR) for the spray rate (S), inlet temperature (T), atomization pressure (A), and percentage of coating (P). The batches from Trials 3 and 4 combined gave her 52 kg of uncoated tablets. She planned to use 9 kg of uncoated tablets for the trials to establish PAR. Rao proposed a five-trial optimal design to accommodate the available quantity of tablets. Optimal designs are experimental designs where trials are selected to optimize a statistical criterion of interest. The criterion is usually chosen based on a predetermined model. In the case of the commonly used D-optimal designs, the generalized variances of the model parameter estimates are minimized. This model dependence, which requires selecting a model before starting the experimentation, has been the main criticism of the use of optimal designs, mainly when the goal of an investigation is exploration and discovery, which implies no prior knowledge of such a model.

Table 8.4 is a five-trial optimal design to justify the proven acceptable ranges for the film-coating process. The primary response of interest was dissolution. Tablet appearance, including twinning, chipping, breakage, logo bridging, and core erosion, was monitored during and after the coating process. Assay and related substances were also tested.

Experimental Data

There were no issues with tablet appearance, the assay was on target, and the related substances were well below the acceptance criteria. Table 8.4 shows the experimental design and percentage dissolved at 30 min Q30.

Table 8.4: A optimal design to justify the proven acceptable ranges for a film-coating process

Trial	Order	S	T	D	P	Q30 %
1	3	+	–	+	–	81
2	4	+	+	–	+	78
3	2	–	–	+	+	75
4	5	–	–	–	–	79
5	1	–	+	+	–	79
	–	25	40	10	2	
	+	50	60	15	4	

S: spray rate, g/min
T: inlet temperature, °C
D: drum speed, rpm
P: percentage of film coating
Q30: percentage dissolved at 30 min

Analysis

The small variation in the Q30 percentages obtained from the experiments in Table 8.4 confirms that the product's quality attributes were consistent across the experimental settings of the coating parameters.

What to do next

The team used the operating ranges in Table 8.4 for future scale-up trials.

Evaluating packaging options

Yesim had to evaluate packaging options in parallel to the process development studies. Previous stability studies indicated that the product was sensitive to moisture because of the amide drug substance. Yesim had to evaluate four packaging options, two strengths, and two excipients. To include multi-level qualitative factors and maintain the useful characteristics of two-level fractional factorial experiments, Rao used a simple coding scheme to convert two columns, P_1 and P_2, in a 2^{4-1} design into a single column, Packaging, for a four-level factor:

P_1	P_2	Packaging
–	–	Bottle with desiccant, BD
+	–	Desiccant-lined blisters, BLD
–	+	Bottle, B
+	+	Blister, BL

Table 8.5 outlines the 2^{4-1} design to evaluate the packaging options.

Experimental Data

The film-coated tablets were packaged in the packaging options, stored at 40°C/75%RH, and analyzed after 6 months.

Table 8.5: A 2^{4-1} design evaluates packaging options for the product with a moisture-sensitive drug substance.

Trial	Order		P_1	P_2	S	G (P_1P_2S)	%RS
1	4	BD	–	–	–	–	0.23
2	8	BLD	+	–	–	+	0.05
3	7	B	–	+	–	+	0.73
4	2	BL	+	+	–	–	0.40
5	3	BD	–	–	+	+	0.19
6	1	BLD	+	–	+	–	0.08
7	5	B	–	+	+	–	0.80
8	6	BL	+	+	+	+	0.35

%RS is percentage of related substances

Analysis

The normal plot in Figure 8.4 indicates that the packaging configuration seems to control the percentage of related substances in the tablets by minimizing the available moisture.

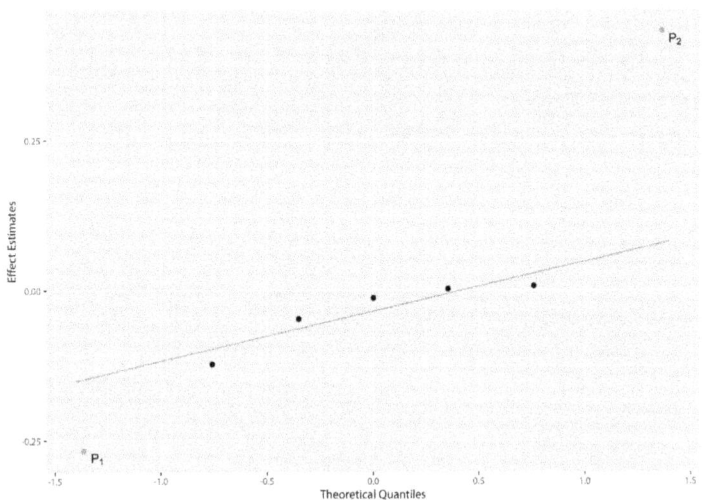

Figure 8.4: The normal plot of the effects for percentage of related substances %RS on stability shows the packaging for the drug product P_1P_2 seems to affect the %RS. The objective of the study was to evaluate the packaging options for a moisture-sensitive drug.

The 2^{4-1} design in Table 8.4 becomes a replicated design for the two factors representing the packaging options:

Packaging			
	P_1	P_2	%RS
Bottle, B	–	+	0.73, 0.80
Blister, BL	+	+	0.40, 0.35
Bottle with desiccant, BD	–	–	0.23, 0.19
Desiccant-lined blister, BLD	+	–	0.05, 0.08

Interpretation

The desiccant-lined blister was most effective because each blister cavity contained a desiccant, resulting in a high capacity to absorb available moisture. The bottle with the one desiccant canister was also acceptable since the percentage of degradant was less than 0.30% and was qualified at 0.43% in toxicology studies. This was important since bottles and blisters were needed to serve different geographical markets.

What to do next

Future studies and the commercial product would use bottles with desiccants or desiccant-lined blisters as needed.

The process development team discussed:

- Additional trials to establish proven acceptable ranges for the various processing steps.
- Documenting critical material attributes, critical quality attributes, and critical process parameters.
- Activities for commercial transfer.
- Bulk hold time studies.
- Justifying the number of process performance qualification batches based on the raw material, the principle of operations of the equipment from laboratory scale to commercial scale, the product development studies, the critical quality attributes, the clinical manufacturing campaigns, and the process knowledge gained during development.

If you wondered

John's three-quarter experimental design layout for four factors (A, B, C, D) in 12 trials

Trial	A	B	C	D	ABCD
1	−	+	−	−	−
2	−	−	+	−	−
3	−	−	−	+	−
4	−	+	+	+	−
5	+	−	−	−	−
6	+	+	+	−	−
7	+	+	−	+	−
8	+	−	+	+	−
9	−	−	−	−	+
10	−	+	+	−	+
11	−	+	−	+	+
12	−	−	+	+	+

For this design, using Trials 1 through 8 only, we can estimate the main effects of A, B, C, and D free from confounding with any two-factor interactions. Assuming that interactions involving three or more factors are negligible, this gives us the main effect estimates free from confounding with interaction effects. We can similarly estimate the two-factor interactions AB, AC, and AD using Trials 5 through 12. Finally, we can estimate the remaining two-factor interactions, BC, BD, and CD, using Trials 1 through 4 and 9 through 12. We should also note that this design can be blocked into two unequal blocks using ABCD as the block generator. In this scheme, the first eight trials and the last four trials, respectively, will constitute the two blocks.

We can also block this design into two equal-size blocks using AB interaction. Further blocking schemes of this design can be found in John (1964). As noted by John, for 10 or 11 factors, it is preferable to use the 12-trial Plackett and Burman design, which gives orthogonal effects and uses all 12 trials to estimate the effects.

A partial list of visual defects for tablets:

Uncoated	Broken, split, chipped, capped, specks, mottled, a surface defect due to sticking or picking, legibility issues with debossed characters, and foreign particles.
Coated	Broken, chipped, sticky, twinned, tablet core erosion, capped, specks, agglomerated tablets, color variation, absence of color, rough surface, legibility issues with debossed characters, and foreign particles.

NOTES

Ankenman, B. (1999). Design of experiments with two-level and four-level factors. *Journal of Quality Technology* 31(4): 363–375. Provides two-level and four-level factorial designs for practitioners.

Box, M.J., and Draper, N.R. (1971). Factorial designs, the |X'X| criterion, and some related matters. *Technometrics* 4(13): 731–742.

Bradley, J. and Montgomery, D. (2019). *Design of Experiments: A Modern Approach*. New York: Wiley.

Burdick, R., LeBlond, D.J., Quiroz J., Sidor, L, Vukovinsky, K., and Zhang, L. (2017). *Statistical Applications for Chemistry Manufacturing and Controls (CMC) in the Pharmaceutical Industry*. Switzerland: Springer.

John, P.W.M. (1964). Blocking of $3(2^{n-k})$ designs, *Technometrics* 6(4): 371–376.

John, P.W.M. (1971). *Statistical Design and Analysis of Experiments.* New York: Wiley.

No technique or tools can replace technical expertise. The goal is to integrate technical knowledge and statistical tools to solve problems.

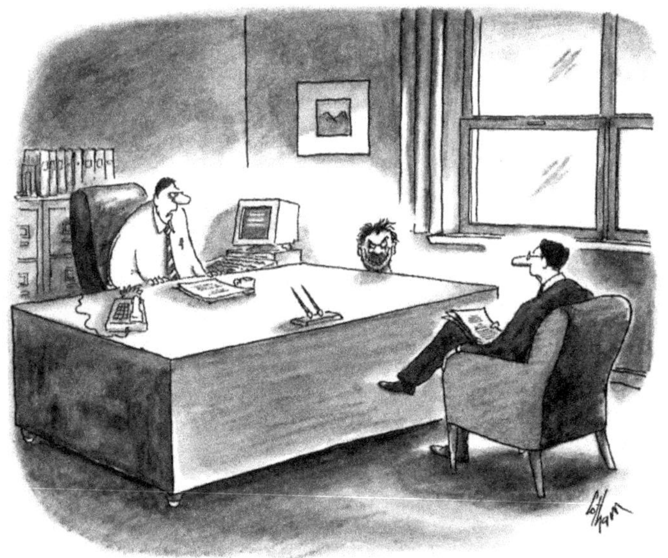

"As soon as one problem is solved, another rears its ugly head."

9

How Does Experimental Design Enable Problem-Solving?

This chapter shows the versatility of experimental design thinking in addressing problems. Three approaches are outlined below.

- Picking the winner: Sometimes, the experimenter wants to know which factor settings will give them the required response. Experimental design thinking can provide a structured approach with which to address the issue.
- Updating our inferences: Resource constraints force experimenters to do two or three experiments in the hope of learning or judging what to do next. In the early development stages, tools like factorial-one-factor-at-a-time plans and Bisgaard plots help experimenters reason with the data using prior knowledge and deciding what to do next.

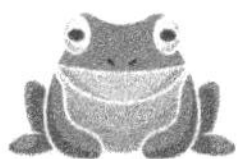

- Finding a resolution: Investigators routinely use experimental design thinking to identify root causes or catalyze the discovery of a solution.

Picking the winner

Identifying a powder in a bottle formulation for a preclinical study

Problem

The formulator had limited drug substance to conduct three trials at an early preclinical stage. The drug substance was susceptible to oxidation, and the formulator had to evaluate three excipients and three antioxidants (G, A, C). Ott's screening design was used in this case.

Design, Data, Analysis, and Decision

Table 9.1 outlines Ott's screening design with the initial percentage of related substance data and the data after storing the samples for 2 weeks at 50°C/80%RH. The data patterns are matched to the column signs. The combination of excipients and the antioxidant in Trial 1 gave the lowest percentage of related substances and was chosen as the formulation for the early preclinical studies. This approach is recommended with caution because it assumes no interactions between the formulation components and depends on the team's prior knowledge.

Table 9.1: Using Ott's screening design to identify excipients for a preclinical formulation. Samples were stored for 2 weeks at 50°C/80%RH.

Trial	DS	Solvent	Cosolvent	Diluent	G	A	C	% Related Substances	
								Initial	2 weeks
1	+	+	+	–	+	–	–	0.11	0.19
2	+	+	–	+	–	+	–	0.09	1.27
3	+	–	+	+	–	–	+	0.13	0.50

Setting up an encapsulation machine

Problem

The facility had an encapsulation machine with four dosing pins that sequentially tamped the powder in the body of the capsule shell. The pins could be set at different heights to accommodate the amount of powder in a particular capsule size. The operators would spend time adjusting the pins by trial and error until the target weight for the capsule was achieved. Over time this became the domain expertise of two operators who had a "feel" for the machine. While the two operators gained implicit knowledge, the machine could only be used when at least one of them was present at the facility.

Both operators were absent during a clinical manufacturing campaign using the encapsulation machine. The other operators at the facility used design thinking to identify the settings of the tamping pins during the setup phase of the manufacturing. The pins were assumed to be factors, and a two-level 2^{4-1} design was outlined and executed.

Design, Data, Analysis, and Decision

Table 9.2 shows the 2^{4-1} experimental layout and the data where 10 capsules were collected at each setting for measuring the weight of capsules filled with the blend. The target fill weight of 10 Size 4 capsules was 2000 mg ± 100 mg. The average weight of 10 empty Size 4 capsules is 47 mg. The procedure was to collect 10 capsules, record the individual weight of five capsules, and record the total weight of the 10 capsules. The pin settings are unitless.

Table 9.2: A 2^{4-1} design to identify the pin height settings in an encapsulation machine

Trial	Order	Pin 1	Pin 2	Pin 3	Pin 4	Weight of 10 capsules, mg
1	7	–	–	–	–	1935.4
2	8	+	–	–	+	2062.7
3	3	–	+	–	+	2074.8
4	6	+	+	–	–	2010.1
5	2	–	–	+	+	2093.4
6	9	+	–	+	–	2045.3
7	4	–	+	+	–	2058.2
8	1	+	+	+	+	Pounding
	–	13	13	13	13	
	+	18	18	18	18	

The dosing pin settings from Trial 4 in Table 9.2 were chosen to encapsulate the rest of the blend because the weight of 10 capsules was closest to the target of 2000 mg. To validate this choice, the operators collected 10 capsules every 10 min of the production. The total weight of each sample of 10 capsules is given in Table 9.3. As seen in the line plot, the total weight of a sample of 10 capsules remained well within the target fill weight of 2000 ± 100mg.

Table 9.3: Total weight of 10 capsules collected at 10-min intervals during the encapsulation process

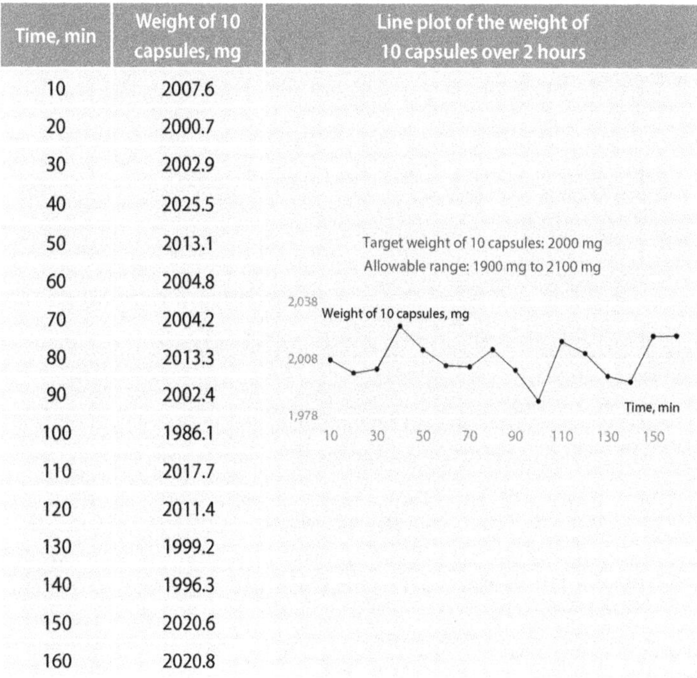

Time, min	Weight of 10 capsules, mg	Line plot of the weight of 10 capsules over 2 hours
10	2007.6	
20	2000.7	
30	2002.9	
40	2025.5	
50	2013.1	
60	2004.8	
70	2004.2	
80	2013.3	
90	2002.4	
100	1986.1	
110	2017.7	
120	2011.4	
130	1999.2	
140	1996.3	
150	2020.6	
160	2020.8	

Updating our inferences

Deciding on a salt form and identifying excipient ratios

Problem

After a molecule was nominated for development, early synthesis work had to rely on one of two salt forms, followed by identifying the temperature and excipient ratios for a stable formulation of the selected salt form.

Design, Data, Analysis, and Decision

Drawing a simple decision tree was the first step in outlining the problem.

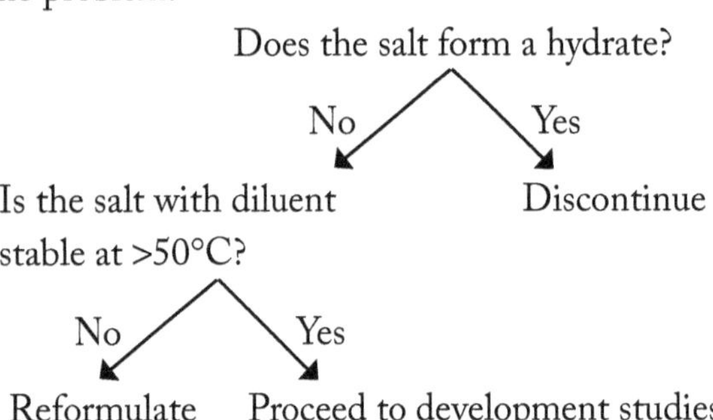

Next, the formulators used factorial one-factor-at-a-time experiments to decide (see Daniel, 1994).

Step 1: Does the salt form a hydrate?

The chemist synthesized enough drug substance of the two salts to do two trials each. The temperature and the ratio of drug substance to diluents were maintained at settings the chemist used as starting levels. The two experiments shown in Table 9.4 show that Form 1 does not form a hydrate, and the total percentage of related substances was less than 0.2%.

Table 9.4: Identifying the salt form

Trial	Form	Temp	Ratio	% Moisture		% Related substances	
				Measured	Difference	Measured	Difference
1	–	–	–	0.41		0.11	
2	+	–	–	8.31	7.90	0.72	0.61
–	1	30°C	0.5:1				
+	2	Not applicable	Not applicable				

Step 2: Are the chosen salt form and excipient ratios stable at 50°C?

The chemist synthesized enough of Salt Form 1 to conduct three trials. The difference columns show no effect of the temperature or the excipients ratio on the percentages of moisture or related substances. The next step was to develop the solution formulation for preclinical studies using Salt Form 1.

Table 9.5: Effect of temperature and excipients on the stability of Salt Form 1

				% Moisture		% Related substances	
Trial	Form	Temp	Ratio	Measured	Difference	Measured	Difference
3	–	–	–	0.35		0.12	
4	–	+	–	0.29	-0.06	0.16	0.04
5	–	+	+	0.28	-0.01	0.18	0.02
–	1	30	0.5:1				
+	Not applicable	50	1:1				

Using the Bisgaard plot to identify the diluent(s) to avoid

Problem

After completing a 2^{4-1} design to evaluate the effect of excipients on the stability of the formulation, the normal plot shown in Figure 9.1 suggested none of the excipients affected the stability. The experimenters disagreed with the conclusion from the normal plot because the related substances had increased at least twice the initial value after 6 weeks of storage at 50°C/80%RH.

Design, Data, Analysis, and Decision

Table 9.6: A 2^{4-1} design to study the effect of excipients on the drug product stability. The average initial percentage of related substances (%RS) was 0.182%. The samples were stored for 6 weeks at 50°C/80%RH

Trial	Order	P	L	DT	D	%RS after 6 weeks
1	7	–	–	–	–	0.783
2	8	+	–	–	+	0.408
3	3	–	+	–	+	0.432
4	6	+	+	–	–	0.579
5	2	–	–	+	+	0.519
6	9	+	–	+	–	0.562
7	4	–	+	+	–	0.606
8	1	+	+	+	+	0.455
	–	MC	SA	ST	DCP	
	+	HPC	GB	CP	TCP	

P: polymer (MC: methylcellulose, HPC: hydroxypropyl cellulose)
L: lubricant (SA: stearic acid, GB: glyceryl behenate)
DT: disintegrant (ST: starch, CP: crospovidone)
D: diluent (DCP: dicalcium phosphate, TCP: tricalcium phosphate)

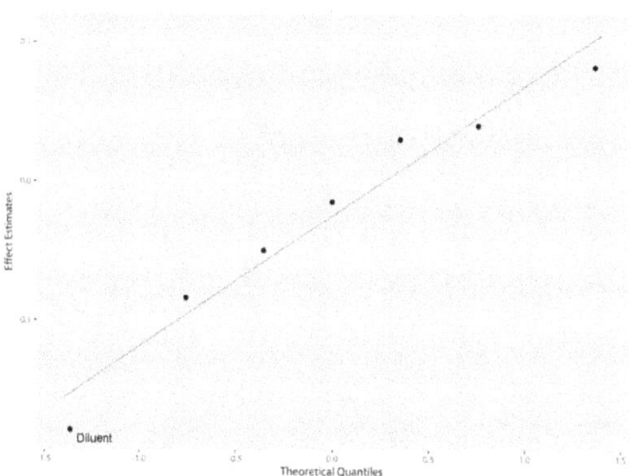

Figure 9.1: The normal plot of effects for percentage of related substances shows the excipients did not affect the product stability after 6 weeks of storage at 50°C/80%RH. "Diluent" is highlighted because further investigation indicated it influenced the stability.

During the discussions on the data, the analytical chemist said the range of five measurements was 0.20%, and the chemical development scientist indicated their range of five measurements was 0.28%. Five preparations of the same sample were measured. The range here is the difference between the highest and lowest measurements within the five samples. Such differences between functional groups within CMC are not unusual during the early development stages. Since all the readings after 6 weeks were at least twice the initial reading, the conclusion that none of the excipients had a significant effect on the stability of the drug product was suspected.

The statistician used the ranges the analytical chemist and the chemical development scientist provided to generate a Bisgaard plot (Figure 9.2.)

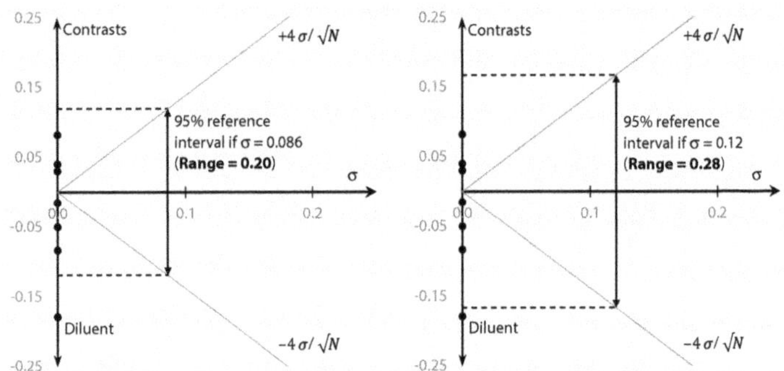

Figure 9.2: Bisgaard plots using 0.20% and 0.28% as ranges to identify diluents influencing the stability of the drug product.

The Bisgaard plot (also known as the conditional inference chart) uses prior knowledge of error to explore which factors could be active in small two-level experiments and provides the experimenter with plausible interpretations. It is a hypothesis generation tool. The standard deviation σ in Figure 9.2 is calculated by dividing the range by a constant for a sample size of 5. Here we have a standard deviation of 0.086 for the left panel of Figure 9.2 and a standard deviation of 0.12 for the right panel of Figure 9.2 (see "If you wondered," p. 175, for further explanation of the Bisgaard plot.)

The Bisgaard plots in Figure 9.2 show that the two diluents have different effects on percentage of related substances after 6 weeks of storage at 50°C/80%RH. The analytical chemist suggested the differing basic properties between the diluents may have been responsible for the effect of the diluents. The team set up three trials to confirm the suggestion.

Trial	Experiments	Initial pH	Initial %RS	%RS after 72 hours
1	Drug substance + 15% water	1.6	0.178	0.259
2	Drug substance + Diluent 1 + 15% water	7.4	0.234	1.187
3	Drug substance + Diluent 2 + 15% water	6.3	0.278	0.799

Based on the results from the three trials, the experimenters decided to replace the basic diluent with a slightly acidic diluent and reformulate the tablet. The experimenters successfully formulated a tablet product using P+, L-, DT+, and a somewhat acidic diluent. The percentage of related substances for this product was 0.27% after 6 months of storage at 40°C/75%RH, which was within the toxicologically qualified limit of 0.36%.

Finding a solution

Resolving the issue in a clinical batch investigation

Identifying systematic errors associated with materials, methods, machines, personnel, and measurement can be challenging and takes considerable detective work. Experimental designs to address questions concerning material, methods, machines, personnel, and measurements could reduce uncertainty from systematic errors.

Partial knowledge about our systems is expressed in the form

$$y = f(x_k) + e(x_u)$$

where $x_k = (x_{k1}, x_{k2}, \ldots, x_{kn})$ are known explanatory factors or variables, and e is a function of $x_u = (x_{u1}, x_{u2}, \ldots)$ where x_u's represent unknown variables or factors influencing the process. What we call random error e is due to unaccounted-for causes. The goal of the investigation is to identify factors in the unknown e box and move them to the known x_k box:

$$y = f(x_k) + e(x_u)$$

Problem

The blend uniformity analysis (BUA) from a 70 kg Phase 3 clinical supply batch (Lot DCP107) had a average assay of 91.7% with a 9.5% relative standard deviation (RSD). It failed the acceptance criteria of 95%–105% mean blend assay with less than 5% RSD. Four previous drug product lots of the 0.7 mg strength tablet had a average BUA assay value ranging from 98% to 103%, with RSD values ranging from 0.4% to 2.7%.

An investigation was undertaken to understand the factors causing the BUA failure.

Design, Data, Analysis, and Decision

The investigation of root causes began with a detailed discussion between the operators and the analytical chemist. Figure 9.3 shows their output.

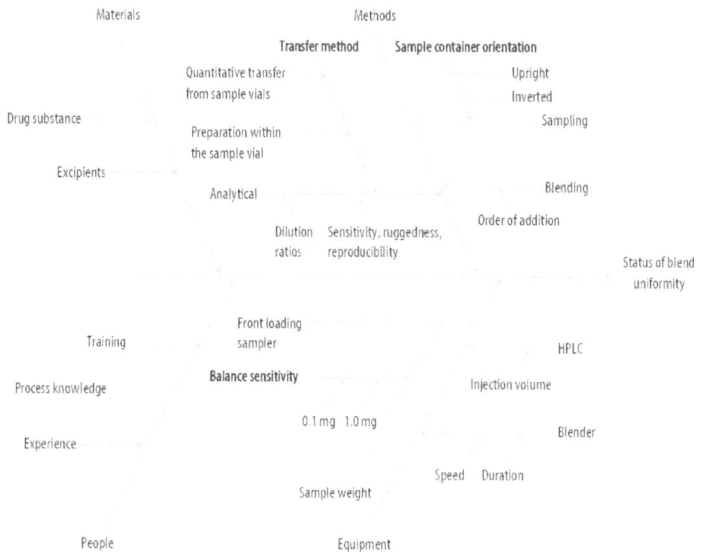

Figure 9.3: Output from the detailed discussion to identify factors affecting the status of the blend. The team decided to evaluate the effect of the balance sensitivity, transfer method, and sample container orientation on the assay's average and standard deviation values.

Two operators were involved in this process: Operator 1 sampled the blend, and Operator 2 took care of the post-sampling details, including sending the samples for analysis. Operator 2 placed the sample bottles in a plastic bag for submission to the analytical chemist. The sample handling procedures did not specify the sample container orientation during storage. The analytical chemist who prepared and analyzed the sample using high-performance liquid chromatography (HPLC) also had been recently trained. According to the analytical procedure, the analyst made a quantitative transfer from the original sample container to the analytical vial for sample preparation.

Based on the above, they investigated sample handling, including balance sensitivity, transfer method, and sample container orientation, using a 2^3 factorial design as outlined in Table 9.7.

- The two levels for balance sensitivity were 0.1 mg and 1.0 mg.
- The two levels for the transfer method included the analyst preparing the sample in the 60 cc amber glass bottles containing the blend sample or making a quantitative transfer of the desired blend weight to another 60 cc amber vial before sample preparation.
- The two levels for sample orientation were keeping the closed amber glass vials with the powder blend upright or inverted for 24 hours. For the inverted samples where the sample preparation was within the amber glass vial, a portion of the solvent was used to rinse the bottle cap and extract any residual drug product.

The operators blended a 12 kg batch in a 24 L bin blender using a process similar to the process used with the clinical supplies batch. The operators used a surrogate drug substance with similar physical characteristics to the much more expensive drug substance used in Lot DCP107. The blend was sampled from distinct locations in the bin blender using a front-loading sampler that dispensed the samples directly into a vial. The sample weight was three times the tablet weight. The data is presented in Table 9.7.

Table 9.7: A 2^3 design to study the effect of sample container orientation and transfer method on the average blend uniformity assay and standard deviation

Trial	Order	Balance sensitivity	Transfer method	Sample container orientation	Average assay (n = 10)	s[a]	Log (s + 1)	RSD[b]
1	5	–	–	–	100.0	0.60	0.20	0.60
2	4	+	–	–	99.8	1.23	0.35	1.23
3	1	–	+	–	97.2	0.59	0.20	0.61
4	3	+	+	–	96.6	1.75	0.44	1.81
5	7	–	–	+	96.0	6.25	0.86	6.51
6	6	+	–	+	94.9	8.42	0.97	8.87
7	8	–	+	+	92.5	1.68	0.43	1.81
8	2	+	+	+	92.2	1.49	0.40	1.62
	–	0.1 mg	No transfer[c]	Upright				
	+	1 mg	Quantitative transfer[d]	Inverted				

[a]Standard deviation;

[b]Relative standard deviation;

[c]No transfer: Sample preparation is in the same bottle that contained the blend sample. The sample weight was 300 mg;

[d]Transfer: Sample preparation is in a new bottle after transferring 200 mg from the original container.

The normal plot of the effects in Figure 9.4 shows that the transfer method and sample container orientation (two of the three factors) seem to influence the average blend assay value. Further statistical analysis shows that these two effects are indeed significant (see "If you wondered," p. 175.)

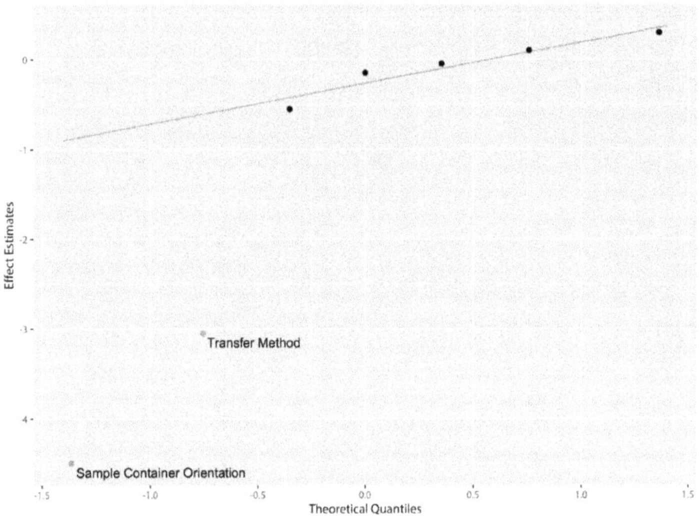

Figure 9.4: The normal plot of effects for average blend assay (n = 10) shows that the transfer method and sample container orientation seem to affect the blend uniformity analysis assay.

Since balance sensitivity is not a significant factor for the average percentage of blend assay, the 2^3 design in Table 9.7 projects to a 2^2 design replicated twice as shown by the cube and square plots. The arrow in the square plot points to the preferred post-handling conditions for blend samples—keeping the sample container upright and preparing the sample within the sample container.

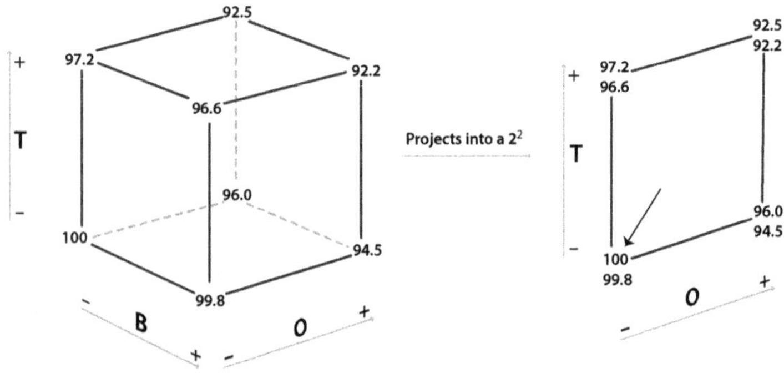

To determine which factor influences the variability, we can use the sample variance or sample standard deviation for the same design rather than the average. In such cases, we often use the log transformation of the sample standard deviation, which is half of the log-transformed sample variance, to better approximate normal distribution. In this case, since some estimates of the standard deviation were less than one in magnitude, we consider the log(s+1) as the response (Table 9.7) to see the effect of the factors on the variability in the measurements within 10 samples. The normal plot of the log(s+1) in Figure 9.5 for the percentage of assay values shows the sample container orientation seems to affect the variability of the assay values. An inverted sample container contributes to assay variability because the material can be unevenly trapped in the cap liner or the lip of the amber glass vial and is not entirely extracted during the sample preparation.

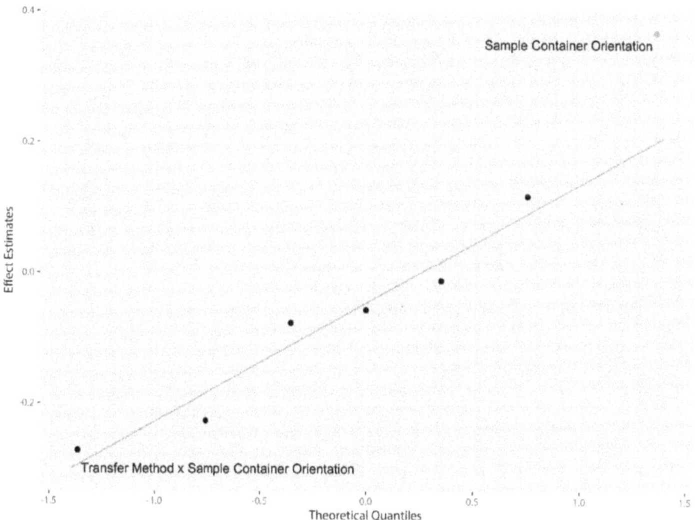

Figure 9.5: The normal plot of effects for log (standard deviation +1) of the blend assay showing the sample container orientation seems to affect the variability of the assay values. Transfer method x sample container orientation is highlighted because it has practical importance, as explained in the text.

In studying Figure 9.5 (see the interaction term transfer method x sample container orientation) and Trials 5 and 6 in Table 9.7, the experimenter reasoned there might be an interaction effect between the sample container orientation and the transfer method, which could be practically important. The interaction plot in Figure 9.6 shows the variability (log(s+1)) is low when the sample container is inverted or upright, and there is a quantitative transfer. The variability (log(s+1)) is higher when the sample container is inverted and the analytical sample preparation is within the sample container. But, if the container is kept upright, the variability (log(s+1)) seems to be insensitive to the transfer method. The cause of the higher variation for the inverted sample container could be loss due to adherence of the blended powder to the sample container closure and the incomplete extraction of the powder blend from the sample container closure.

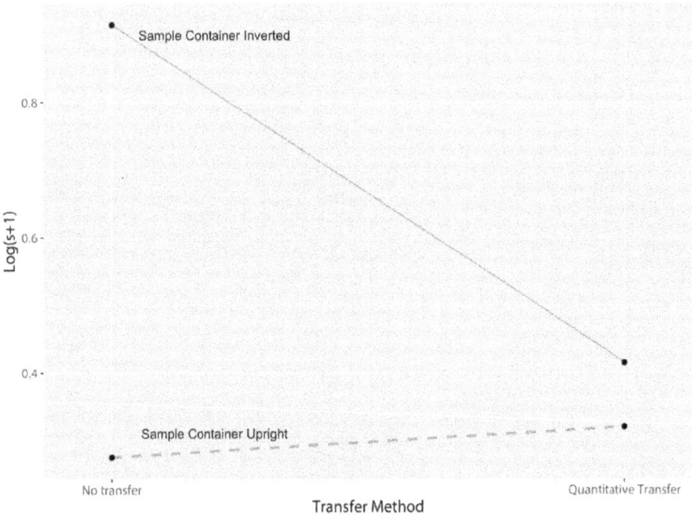

Figure 9.6: The plot indicates a potential interaction between the transfer method and the sample container orientation for log(s+1).

An aside

The normal plot of the effects did not imply a statistically significant interaction between the orientation and the transfer method. Yet the interaction plot in Figure 9.6 hints at possible interaction. While this is thought-provoking, the interaction plot does not necessarily imply a statistically significant effect. For illustration, we consider a model for log(s+1) with sample container orientation and its interaction with the transfer method. The ANOVA for this model, given below, shows the interaction is not statistically significant at a 5% significance level ($p<0.05$) but is statistically significant at a 10% significance level ($p<0.1$). For a conservative analysis, we employ a 5% level, while for exploratory analysis, we can employ a 10% level. Experimenters accept a more significant chance of a false alert at a 10% level. The interaction between the transfer method and the sample container orientation also has a practical explanation.

However, we confirm exploratory findings in follow-up experiments in product development. We recommend not using *p*-values mechanically to decide what effects are significant and what effects to ignore. Graphical methods provide increased insights by enabling information in the data and the experimenter's mind to interact effectively.

	Sum of squares	Degrees of freedom	Mean squares	F-ratio	*p*-value
Orientation	0.2701	1	0.2701	9.000	0.03
Transfer Method × Orientation	0.1485	1	0.1485	4.948	0.08
Error	0.1501	5	0.0300		
Total	0.5687	7			

We consider another angle to discuss the *p*-value cut-off. ANOVA and the normal plot of the effects compare the presumably significant effects against the leftover effects deemed insignificant. These make up the error term. Intuitively, the more effects set aside as insignificant, the easier it is to compare the potentially significant effects against them. Simplistically, we can see this in the line we draw on a normal plot of the effects. It is simpler to "secure" a line against which the remaining effects are tested as more effects are grouped as nonsignificant. There is not much difference between having one effect (orientation) in the model against six effects in the error term or two effects in the model against five effects in the error term. Therefore, it is acceptable to include a borderline significant second effect in the model for further testing using ANOVA. We caution readers that as the ratio between the number of effects in the model and the number of effects in the errors gets larger, we will quickly reach a point where testing is unreliable.

Back to the problem

The operators compressed the 12 kg blend using the surrogate drug substance to confirm the blend uniformity analysis results. The average assay of n = 3 tablets from the beginning, middle, and end of the compression ranged from 97.5% to 99.5%, with a 1.4% to 2.5% RSD, reconfirming the blend to be homogenous.

The clinical supply batch was resampled and reanalyzed using these learnings, including a balance with 0.1 mg sensitivity, preparing the sample for HPLC analysis within the container, and keeping the sample container upright. The average percentage of assay was 100.6%, with a 1.3% RSD, within acceptable limits. The blend was compressed, and samples were collected at the beginning, middle, and end of the compression process.

Compression stage	Average assay (n = 3)	Range	RSD
Beginning	98.90	3.1	2.7
Middle	100.7	4.6	1.8
End	99.20	1.5	0.9

The operators and analysts updated their training modules to reflect this learning.

- Use a balance with d = 0.1 mg sensitivity.
- Prepare the sample for analysis in the blend sample container.
- Keep the sample container upright.

The clinical batch (Lot DCP107) and possibly future batches would have been at risk if the process had not been studied and corrected.

A parallel effort to identify a sample handling procedure not reliant on a specific sample container orientation was evaluated. Keeping samples upright is a challenge during transport between and within sites. A system can be robust only when the underlying factors do not affect the quality of the outcome under a wide range of settings.

The powder blend sample in a 10 ml container was weighed on a balance with 0.1 mg sensitivity. All the blend sample powder in the dry state was transferred into the preparatory flask during the sample preparation for analysis. A procedure was outlined to rinse the sample container and the cap with the analytical solvent to extract residual blend powder. The average assay for 10 samples was 100.8%, with a 1.7% RSD. The team decided to implement this procedure for future batches.

Developing a robust particle size analysis method for early development candidates

Problem

Discussing initial particle size specification is complicated when the stakeholders (drug substance, analytical, and drug product) cannot agree on the method that best represents the particle size characteristics. ISO 13320 outlines the challenges regarding particle size measurements using laser diffraction methods. It is difficult to interpret preclinical data and decide on early-phase clinical formulation development when there are differing particle size data from various CMC functions.

A water-soluble compound was entering Phase 2. The drug substance group had made two lots with visually different particle sizes (Table 9.8). They submitted the samples to their drug product and analytical counterparts.

Table 9.8: Qualitative particle size assessment under a polarized light microscope

Lot	Size of >75% of samples in microns	Image	Visual description
A	360	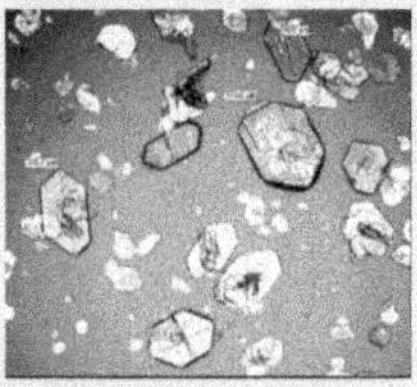	Big
B	40	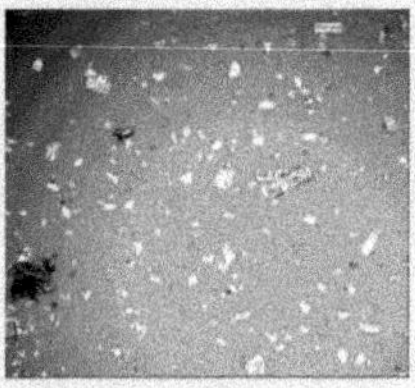	Small

Table 9.9 shows the d_{50} data reported by the various functions. d_{50} and d_{90} are statistical parameters from the cumulative particle size distribution. They indicate the size below which 50% or 90% of all particles are found.

Table 9.9: Drug substance d_{50} particle size for the same lot reported by various functions

Function	Laser diffraction method	Lot A	Lot B
Drug Product	Dry powder. 0.1 bar pressure	198	19
Analytical	A wet method with sonication	56	14
Drug Substance	Dry powder. 3.0 bar pressure	23	8

The drug substance group used a dry powder laser diffraction method at three-bar dispersion pressure; the analytical group used an existing wet method laser diffraction with sonication to disperse agglomerates, and the drug product group used a dry powder laser diffraction method at 0.1 bar dispersion pressure.

The analyst had to develop a robust particle size measurement method representative of the drug substance particle size.

Design, Data, Analysis, and Decision

The analyst used a split-plot design (Table 9.10) to evaluate three whole-plot factors (the two-drug substance lots, the amount of drug substance in a sample, and the sonication time) and one subplot factor (the stirrer speed.) The responses were d_{50} and d_{90} in microns.

Table 9.10: A 2^3 x 2^1 split-plot design to study the effect of measurement factors on drug substance particle size

Trial	Order	Drug substance particle size	Drug substance amount, mg	Sonication time, min	Stirrer speed			
					1000 rpm		2000 rpm	
					d_{50} um	d_{90} um	d_{50} um	d_{90} um
1	8	–	–	–	13	27	13	27
2	3	+	–	–	200	405	179	366
3	4	–	+	–	13	28	13	28
4	5	+	+	–	201	405	218	406
5	6	–	–	+	11	25	12	27
6	1	+	–	+	33	73	38	90
7	7	–	+	+	12	26	11	26
8	2	+	+	+	40	93	40	98
	–	Small	100	0				
	+	Big	200	2				

Figures 9.7 and 9.8 are trellis plots executed as facet plots in the ggplot2 package in R. On comparing the rows in both figures, we do not see a significant change in the lines' slopes or extent, suggesting the stirrer speed (1000 rpm vs. 2000 rpm) does not affect the particle size measurement. Comparing the drug substance amount columns (100 mg vs. 200 mg) shows no significant difference either. Comparing the drug substance particle size (small vs. big) and the sonication time (0 min vs. 2 min) columns indicates they may significantly affect the particle size measurement. The changing slopes of the lines between the columns indicate a potential interaction between drug substance particle size and sonication time. This shows that a sonication time of 2 min breaks the bigger particles and affects the particle size measurement, which suggests that the method is not robust to sonication time.

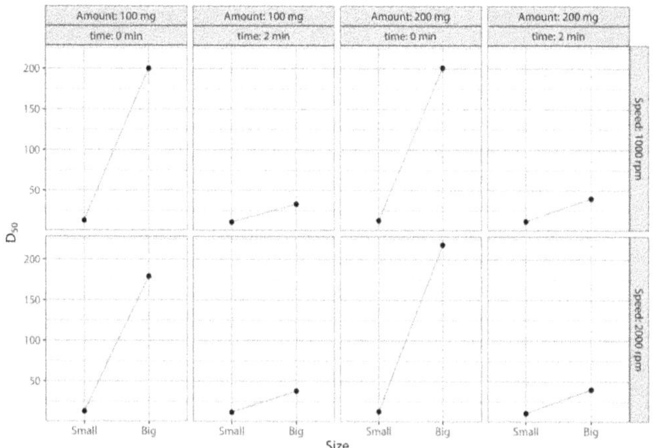

Figure 9.7: The trellis plot shows the effect of qualitative drug substance particle size, sonication time, and their interaction on d_{50}. The line plots indicate the effect of drug substance particle size and sonication time on d_{50}, and the change in slope between the columns means a possible interaction between the two.

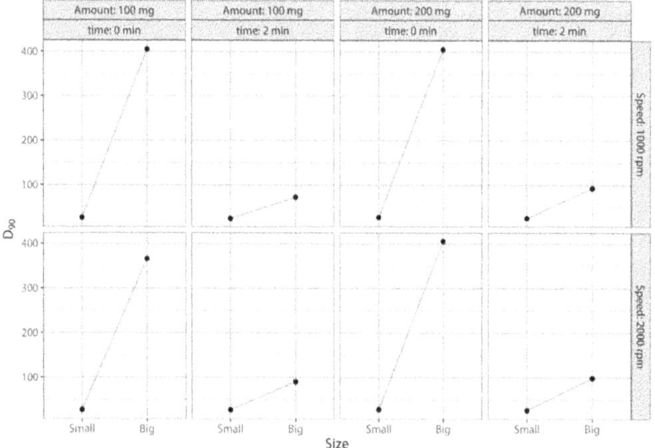

Figure 9.8: The trellis plot shows the effect of qualitative drug substance particle size, sonication time, and their interaction on d_{90}. The line plots indicate the effect of drug substance particle size and sonication time on d_{90}, and the change in slope between the columns means a possible interaction between the two.

The normal plots (Figures 9.9 and 9.10) indicate that the drug substance particle size, sonication time, and an interaction between the drug substance particle size and sonication time may be significant. This is similar to the conclusion from the trellis plots in Figures 9.7 and 9.8. The amount of drug substance and the stirrer speed do not seem to affect the measurement.

Sonication is included to improve dispersion when undispersed agglomerates are visible through microscopy or in the dispersion medium. However, the particle size measurement does not represent the actual particle size if the sonication time breaks up the particles. The intent was to develop a generic particle size measurement technique for early-phase development studies. But, if the measurement technique had been robust, only the drug substance particle size effect should have been significant.

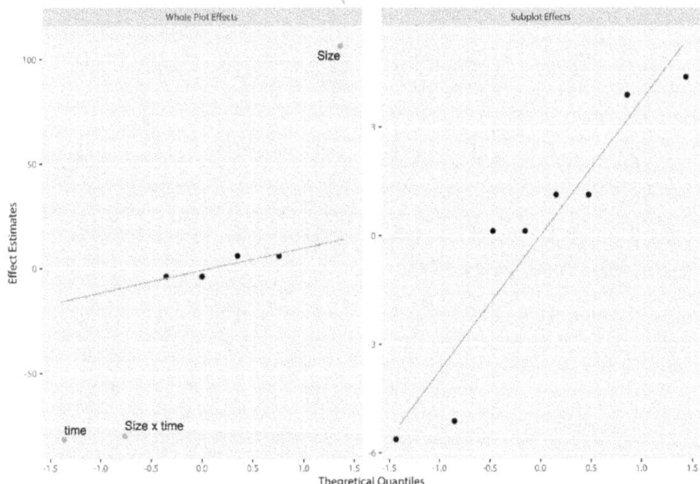

Figure 9.9: The normal plot of the whole-plot effects for d_{50} shows drug substance particle size, sonication time, and interaction between particle size and sonication time may affect d_{50}; the normal plot of the subplot effects for d_{50} shows the effects had no impact on d_{50}.

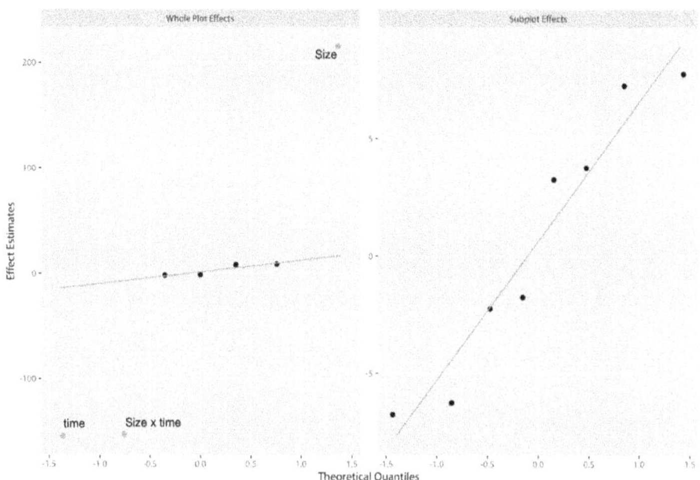

Figure 9.10: The normal plot of the whole-plot effects for d_{90} shows drug substance particle size, sonication time, and interaction between particle size and sonication time may affect d_{90}; the normal plot of the subplot effects for d_{90} shows the effects had no impact on d_{90}.

The analysis prompted the analyst to redesign the sample preparation technique without sonication. The factors studied in the second experimental sequence included the two lots of drug substance, the number of span 85 drops, and the holding time (Table 9.11). Based on Figures 9.7 and 9.8, the analyst decided to fix the sample amount at 150 mg and the stirrer speed at 1500 rpm.

Table 9.11: A 2^3 design to study the effect of qualitative drug substance particle size, the number of span 85 drops, and the holding time on d_{50} and D_{90} particle size using a modified sample preparation technique. The sample size was 150 mg, and the stirrer speed was 1500 rpm

Trial	Order	Drug substance particle size	Number of span 85 drops	Holding time, min	d_{50} um	d_{90} um
1	5	–	–	–	13	29
2	2	+	–	–	214	414
3	8	–	+	–	12	28
4	7	+	+	–	215	404
5	1	–	–	+	13	28
6	3	+	–	+	208	406
7	6	–	+	+	12	28
8	4	+	+	+	218	410
	–	Small	3	0.5		
	+	Big	5	5		

The normal plot in Figure 9.11 shows the drug substance particle size as the only potentially significant effect. This indicates the method may be sensitive to the drug substance particle size, and none of the other factors studied. The analyst developed a robust particle size method for their early development studies. The relevant statistical analysis for some of these conclusions is provided on the book's website, datatodecision.org.

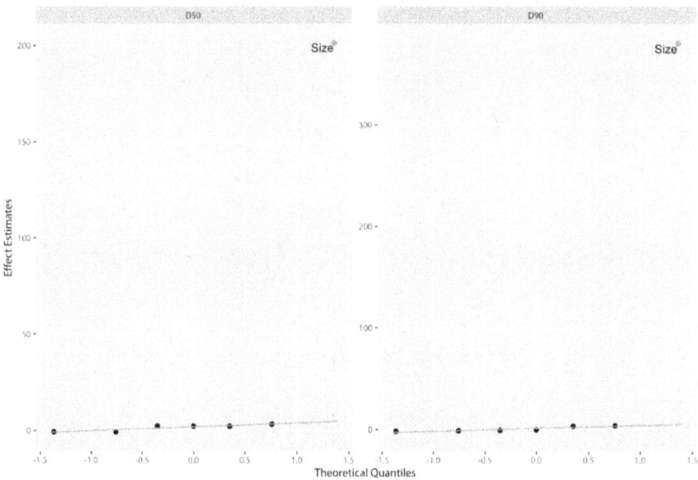

Figure 9.11: The normal plot of the effects for d_{50} and d_{90} using the modified method shows only drug substance particle size may affect d_{50} and d_{90}.

Identifying the process conditions for a target particle size

Problem

A Phase 2 dosage form was a granular powder in a bottle to be reconstituted at the clinic. The product was manufactured using a top-spray fluid-bed granulation process. The formulators needed to identify the formulation and process factors affecting the average granule particle size. They also wanted to know the factor settings that would result in d_{50} particle size between 100 and 200 microns.

Design, Data, Analysis, and Decision

The 2^{5-1} fractional factorial design in Table 9.12 was executed to evaluate the effects of percentage of binder P, the molecular weight of the binder B, atomization pressure A, spray rate S, and inlet temperature T on the granule particle size.

Table 9.12: A 2^{5-1} fractional factorial design to study the effect of binder and fluid-bed processing parameters on the average granule particle size (T = P*B*A*S)

Trial	Order	P	B	A	S	T	d_{50}, µ
1	12	−	−	−	−	+	118
2	15	+	−	−	−	−	35
3	3	−	+	−	−	−	59
4	13	+	+	−	−	+	50
5	1	−	−	+	−	−	134
6	7	+	−	+	−	+	134
7	6	−	+	+	−	+	48
8	16	+	+	+	−	−	78
9	9	−	−	−	+	−	157
10	14	+	−	−	+	+	226
11	10	−	+	−	+	+	172
12	2	+	+	−	+	−	235
13	5	−	−	+	+	+	159
14	11	+	−	+	+	−	254
15	4	−	+	+	+	−	137
16	8	+	+	+	+	+	216

From the normal plot in Figure 9.12 the spray rate S seems to be significant. Moreover, the target d_{50} particle size range was mainly achieved at a high spray rate (Trials 9 to 16).

In Table 9.12, the experimenter noticed the range for Trials 1 to 8 was 35 to 134 microns at S- and Trials 9 to 16 it was 117 to 254 microns at S+. Since the target particle size was 100 to 200 microns, the experimenter analyzed Trials 9 to 16 separately. The normal plot in Figure 9.13 shows the percentage of binder P to be potentially significant. The 2^{4-1} design for Trials 9 to 16 projects to a one-factor design on percentage of binder P. The d_{50} at P– was 137, 157, 159, and 172 microns, and at P+ it was 216, 226, 235, and 254 microns.

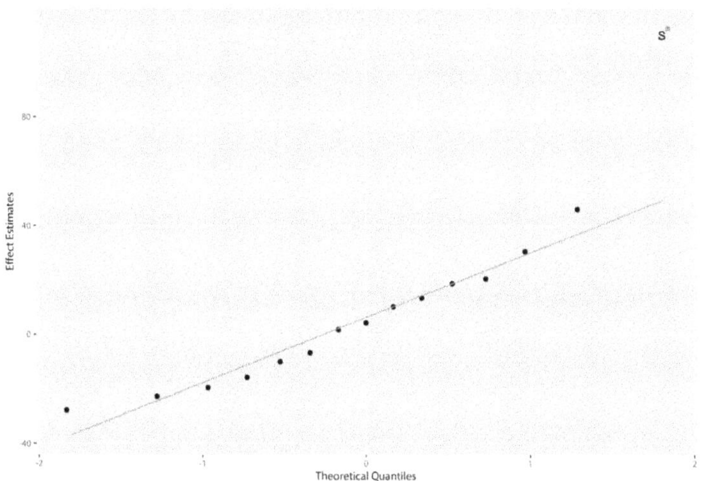

Figure 9.12: The normal plot of the effects for d_{50} granule particle size showing spray rate S may affect the d_{50} granule particle size.

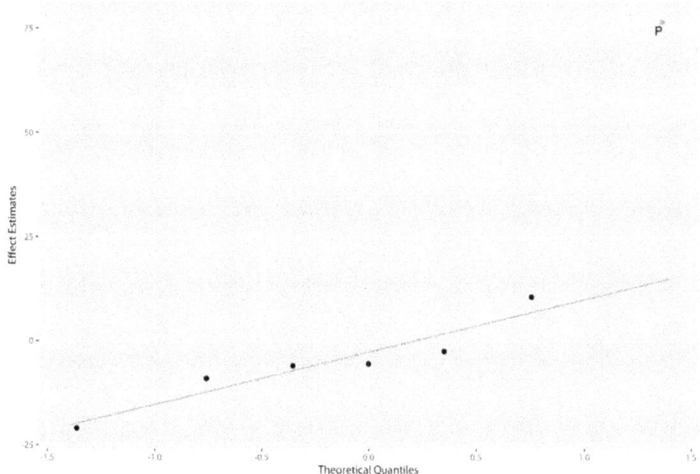

Figure 9.13: The normal plot of the effects analyzing Trials 9 to 16 at the higher spray rate for d_{50} granule particle size shows the percentage of binder P may affect d_{50} granule particle size.

This example reconfirms that the experimenter's critical thinking and active participation are essential components of any statistical and technical analysis. We develop data handling capabilities by not relying on techniques as a substitute for looking at data.

The following settings were chosen to manufacture the clinical lots:

- A low percentage of binder and a high spray rate.
- The low molecular weight binder B and a low atomization pressure A were chosen for operational convenience.
- A high inlet temperature was chosen to minimize the cycle time.

Using these settings [P–, B–, A–, S+, I+], five additional 5 kg clinical lots were successfully manufactured and used in clinical studies. The average particle size for each of the five lots was 148, 159, 158, 163, and 150 microns within the 100 to 200 microns target set by the formulators. The statistical analysis for this example provided on the book's website, datatodecision.org.

If you wondered

Statistical analysis of the clinical batch investigation

The analysis of variance (ANOVA) for the model with only the transfer method and sample container orientation also confirms that the main effects of these factors are significant at the 5% significance level ($p<0.05$). The residual analysis that should follow this ANOVA is provided on the book's website, datatodecision.org.

	Sum of Squares	Degrees of Freedom	Mean Squares	F-ratio	*p*-value
Transfer Method	18.60	1	18.60	108.8	0.00014
Orientation	40.50	1	40.50	236.8	$\sim 2\times10^{-5}$
Error	0.850	5	0.170		
Total	59.95	7			

Early decisions on the manufacturing process with limited data

Compressibility of the drug substance with excipients is essential for tablet manufacturing. The process could be a direct blend, dry granulation, or wet granulation. During the early stages with limited drug substances, manual compression studies assess the drug substance's compressibility and loading.

The flow of powder blends is another essential property of producing tablets, especially when the tablet's drug loading is greater than 5% to 8%. For example, the uniform flow of the powder to fill the tablet die is essential in maintaining weight uniformity. Knowing the flow properties of the powder blend and factors such as particle size and electrostatic forces contributes to stable production. Although imperfect, the Hausner ratio (tap density to bulk density) is easily measured to categorize powder flow.

Using the Bayes theorem and conditional probabilities is helpful when deciding on the manufacturing process for a new drug substance based on limited data.

Bayes's theorem states the following:

$$P(Flows|Compresses) = \frac{P(Compresses|Flows) \times P(Flows)}{P(Compresses)}$$

where P(Flows|Compresses) describes the probability that the blend flows given it compresses.

Based on historical density ratio data, a team had assigned the following probabilities for the blend to flow:

$\frac{\textit{Tap density}}{\textit{Bulk density}}$	P(Flows) %
≤1.35	55
1.36–1.44	40
≥1.45	5

Compresses on a manual machine	P(Compresses), %
Yes	75
No	25
Criteria for "Yes" (manual compression)	
Hardness at two different compression forces	The hardness between the two compression forces is 4 kiloponds apart.
Friability	<1%
Disintegration time	<15 min

A formulation containing 17% drug loading met the compressibility criteria. There was insufficient drug substance to make a 200 g blend for measuring the bulk and tap density. Applying the Bayes theorem, the team calculated their probability in the table below before sufficient drug substance was made to make the required blend amount and measure the density ratio. In the absence of information, they assumed the blend would not flow. Upon receiving sufficient drug substance, they made the blend and measured the tap to bulk density ratio at 1.23. The Bayes formula was updated with this information, as shown in the table below. Knowing the excipients, equipment, processes, and visual observations of the powders, the team decided to move forward with a dry blend followed by compression. Using Bayes thinking with subject matter knowledge is helpful in early decisions regarding the manufacturing process.

Before having the density ratios, %	Event	After having the density ratio, %
5	P(flows)	55
25	P(compresses)	75
25	P(compress|flows)	75
5	P(flows|compresses)	**55**

The Bisgaard Plot

This plot, also called the conditional inference chart, was initially proposed by Bisgaard (1998) for two-level factorial designs as an additional tool to assess the significance of the effects, as in the case of the normal plot of the effects. In a two-level factorial design with N trials, the standard error of the effect estimates is equal to $\frac{2\sigma}{\sqrt{N}}$ where σ is the standard deviation of the experimental error. A rule of thumb is to declare an effect as significant if it is greater than twice its standard error in magnitude, that is, if the effects are beyond the range of $\pm\frac{4\sigma}{\sqrt{N}}$. In the Bisgaard plot, the effect estimates are plotted on the y-axis and the x-axis represents plausible values for σ. The plot also includes two lines indicating the effects are equal to $+\frac{4\sigma}{\sqrt{N}}$ and $-\frac{4\sigma}{\sqrt{N}}$, respectively. Therefore, the distance between these two lines for a given (conjectured) σ also provides the "coverage" for effects that are deemed not significant. Any effect that falls beyond this range is deemed significant.

When converting a range (maximum–minimum) to a measure of dispersion we divide the range by a bias correction factor, d_2. The value of d_2 depends on the sample size, n.

n	2	3	4	5	6	7	8	9	10
d_2	1.128	1.693	2.059	2.326	2.534	2.704	2.847	2.970	3.078

For a given range of 0.5 units and a sample size of six an estimate of the standard deviation will be $\frac{0.5}{2.534} = 0.1973$ units.

The rule of thumb about an effect being deemed significant if its magnitude (absolute value) is twice the error standard deviation implies approximately 5% significance (alpha) under the normality assumption. The reader will recall standard error of the sample mean is standard deviation divided by the square root of the sample size.

NOTES

Banker, G. and Rhodes, C.T. (2002). *Modern Pharmaceutics*. Fourth edition. London: Informa Healthcare.

Bisgaard, S. (1998–99). Conditional inference chart for small unreplicated two-level factorial experiments. *Quality Engineering* 11: 267–271.

Box, G.E.P., Hunter, J.S., and Hunter, W. G. (2005). *Statistics for Experimenters. Design, Innovation, and Discovery.* Second edition. New York: Wiley

Daniel, C. (1994). Factorial one-factor-at-a-time experiments. *The American Statistician* 48(2): 132–135. (Daniel shows how to use design thinking to approach univariate experimentation and still get unbiased estimates of the main effects and interactions using simple subtractions and not evoking matrix computations.)

International Standard. ISO 13320. (1999) *Particle size analysis. Laser diffraction methods – Part 1and 2.* New York: ANSI.

Konstantinos, V.K., Simsek, O., Buckman, M., and Gigerenzer, G. (2020). *Classification in the Wild.* MA: MIT press.

Ott, E., Schilling E., and Neubauer, D.V. (2005). *Process Quality Control. Troubleshooting and Interpretation of Data.* Fourth edition. Wisconsin: ASQ Press.

Snee, R. and Hoerl, R. (2020). *Statistical Thinking: Improving Business Performance.* Third edition. New Jersey: Wiley.

Sometimes we can't see our mistakes until we come out the other side.

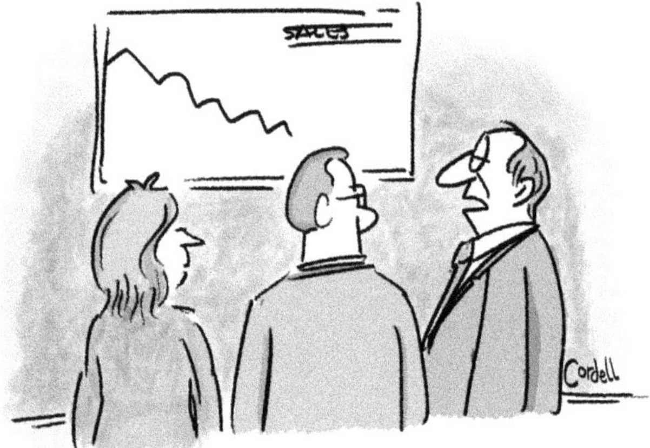

"In hindsight, it was an oversight not to have used foresight."

10

Mistakes Happen

I am positive a doer makes mistakes.

—John Wooden (UCLA basketball coach)

To avoid errors, it is necessary to gain experience; to gain experience it is necessary to make mistakes.

—Peter Lawrence

The reader will note the positivity bias in this book. It makes sense to read a book to learn what works. But by showing what works, we do not mean to create a false sense that anyone who follows the path provided here will develop a useful product. Product developers know that only after the fact does product development appear to be well planned. In fact, it almost always involves improvisation rather than a preordained path to victory. We build the map on our way to creating the product.

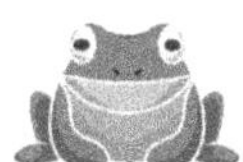

This book has survivorship bias, in that we only show successful case studies. But as experienced experimenters, we have seen more failures than we want to recall. We will highlight some common mistakes made when experimenting. Yesim and Rao do not deny the possibility these are their mistakes.

- Statistical design is no substitute for subject matter knowledge.
- Expect the unexpected: Plan for the plan not going according to the plan.
- Enforce data quality.
- Look beyond the numbers: Avoid the single-number trap.
- A good solution now is better than a perfect one later.
- Anchor your experimental strategy to realities on the ground.
- Use design thinking to strategize resources.
- Experimental design is not just a hypothesis-testing tool.
- *All that is gold does not glitter. Not all who wander are lost.*

—J.R.R. Tolkein

Statistical design is no substitute for subject matter knowledge.

The greatest originality in statistical design and calculations cannot compensate for not knowing a subject, omitting a critical factor, not anticipating likely sources of failure, ignoring the environment, or exploring the wrong design space.

The efforts of William Thompson (Lord Kelvin), the 19th-century British physicist, to calculate the age of the Earth exemplify this principle. Using a thermal gradient approach, he calculated the Earth's age as between 20 million and 100 million years based on the assumption that it had been cooling since it was born. His calculations were spot-on, but he was unaware of convection in the partly fluid interior of the Earth. The deep interior of the Earth provided a large store of heat, which kept the surface temperature gradient high for a long time, and Kelvin's estimate of the age of the Earth was low by a large multiple. Present knowledge indicates the Earth is more than 4 billion years old.

Just as Thompson's calculations were inaccurate because of his lack of knowledge, experiments can fail when we do not account for lurking variables, are absent at the experimental site, or do not anticipate future environments where the data or the experiment will be used.

- Account for lurking variables. A piece of fluid-bed equipment used to produce drug product granulation drew the fluidizing air from outside the facility. The air drawn into the fluid bed was pretreated to keep a humidity level between 35% and 55% relative humidity. Following a 2^{6-2} experimental design, 16 trials using the fluid-bed equipment were completed during the summer months. Analysis revealed that the particle size results fell into two to three groups with high variation in the compressibility data. This was unexpected, and upon further investigation, the experimenters discovered the pretreatment facility had been shut down for repairs halfway through the experiments. The humidity level was high during the summer, and the untreated fluidized air had humidity levels above 70%. The drying time to achieve the desired final moisture content in the product was longer than expected. The increased drying time caused particle attrition, affecting the particle size and the ability to compress tablets. Unfortunately, the experimenter had not used blocking as insurance against such unknowns, and the experimental data could not be used.

- Be present at the experimental site and know your process. Sam, the experimenter, had designed eight experiments using the order suggested by Daniel's one-at-a-time plans. The objective of the trials was to evaluate the effect of temperature, atomization, and spray rate on the granulation particle size, followed by compressibility. Sam did not think it was necessary that he be present during the trial. After the fourth trial, the data showed the atomization pressure and the spray rate did not affect the particle size. This was unexpected since he had varied the two factors over a wide range. When Sam visited the pilot plant during the fifth trial, he saw that most of the atomized and sprayed binder solutions were deposited on the walls and not the product because the available expansion chamber chosen for the trials was too narrow. The experimental effort was discontinued and deemed a failure.
- Anticipate the future context. Every inference is conditional, no matter the experimental design. We cannot assert that other equipment or facilities should behave similarly or differently based on statistical inference alone. Instead, we generalize based on knowledge of the subject and empirical data. This came into play in a process that began with small-scale studies, in which a dosage form did not exhibit any appearance issues at lower equipment speeds. Early formulation compositions did not account for the drug particle size changes in future lots or faster tablet press speeds during scale-up. Upon scaling up, the product failed the acceptable quality levels. The resources needed to reformulate, show formulation equivalence, and update regulatory filing were significant. A model is only as good as the data used to estimate it. If that data does not reflect the future process characteristics, the model may no longer be valid.

- The interaction between design, data analysis, and technical knowledge can enhance practical learning, if not our understanding of the mechanism. In industrial experiments, we aim to find operating conditions under which a process or product can be made with a desired set of qualities. The filtration time when a depolymerized product was emptied into a filtration tank to remove the catalyst varied from 4 hours to 9 hours. Mechanical agitation to force the solvent through the filter medium did not improve the filtration time. The filtration time was the duration from the initial loading of the product into the filter tank to the final emptying of the filter tank. Grace, the plant manager, gathered Janet, the polymer chemist, Carla, the engineer, Ernesto, the statistician, and Joan, the analyst, to improve the filtration process because reducing the variability and the average filtration time would result in cost savings and productivity improvement, which could be redirected to other projects.

The team had two thoughts about the long and variable filtration time:

- After the product was discharged from the reaction vessel into the filtration unit, there may be enough catalysts for residual reactions to be taking place within the filtration unit.
- Highly concentrated pockets of catalyst may be trapped in the polymer, contributing to the variability.

The team suggested a decantation procedure to address the issue. The decantation procedure could be done offline without contributing to the cycle time. The six trials with the decantation procedure showed no improvement in the filtration time (3.5 hours to 7.5 hours.)

The team studied the decantation process at a laboratory scale. They evaluated two conditions:

- Allow the product to settle before removing the supernatant.
- Allow the product to settle, remove the supernatant, and add additional water to quench any residual reaction.

Joan suggested measuring the conductivity of the supernatant during both procedures to monitor catalyst activity as an indirect measure of catalyst concentration. Adding additional water reduced the conductivity significantly compared to not adding extra water.

- The filtration time varied from 1.0 hour to 3.5 hours when the team allowed the product to settle before removing the supernatant.
- When the team allowed the product to settle before removing the supernatant and added extra water to reduce the conductivity significantly, the filtration time varied from 0.33 to 3.0 hours. After some deliberation, Janet wondered if Joan could measure the density of the supernatant from each trial. On reviewing Joan's density measurements Janet found a relation between the density of the supernatant and the filtration time. On reviewing the laboratory records, Janet, Carla, and Ernesto saw the filtration time was less than an hour when they added the additional water quickly, and the density of the supernatant was low. Ernesto pointed out it could be a function of the water addition rate and the quick removal of the supernatant.

Given the urgency of the issue, Grace asked the team to conduct the confirmatory trials in the plant before pursuing additional laboratory experiments to understand the mechanism. Janet, Carla, Joan, and Ernesto calculated the rate of addition, removal, and amount of extra water for the plant trials. The plant ran 12 full-scale trials where the filtration time varied between 2.5 and 4.3 hours. The stable process enabled effective resource planning, and Grace could redirect the cost savings to other projects.

In development, confirmation of results from exploratory work comes from replication, reproducibility, and subject matter knowledge rather than statistical significance.

Amy Hwang captures how perspective can affect your impression of what you're seeing in her *New Yorker* cartoon. Thus it is important to have subject matter knowledge when interpreting results:

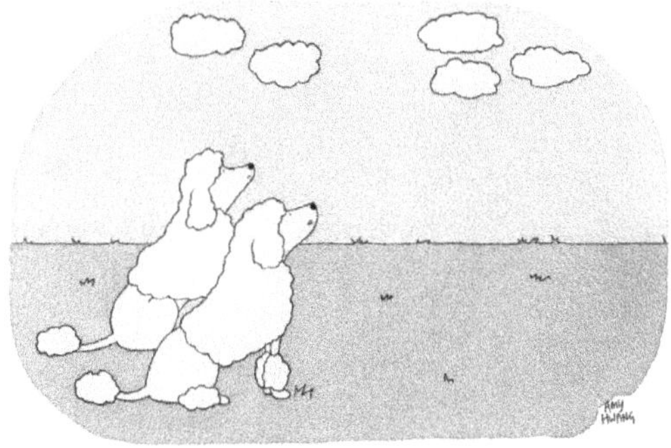

"They all look like ankles."

Expect the unexpected: Plan for the plan not going according to the plan.

Experience has taught us that things often do not go exactly as planned, and thus we must plan for that. In the instances below, things did not go as the researcher expected but they were able to salvage the situation.

- Dan, the statistician, discussed with his team the experiments to evaluate the effect of formulation components and process parameters on product performance, including dissolution and stability. Initially, the team identified nine factors to be investigated, but eliminated two through discussion. Dan initially thought of a 2^{7-4} fractional factorial design with only eight experiments. But he also knew that if the team changed their minds at the last minute and reintroduced the two additional factors for evaluation, the 2^{7-4} design would not accommodate nine factors in eight experiments. Instead, he planned for a 12-trial Plackett and Burman design (also refer to example in "Enforce data quality.") Indeed, just a few days before starting the trials, Rahim, the formulator, asked Dan if one of the two omitted factors could be accommodated in the existing design matrix without changing the number of trials. Since Dan had decided on a 12-trial Placket Burman design using only seven of the 11 columns available, he could easily accommodate the additional factor in one of the four available columns without issue.

- In developing a controlled release product with a target in vitro release profile, the operators had to apply two polymers sequentially, Polymer P1 followed by Polymer P2. Sandra, the formulator, outlined a 2^{5-2} design to evaluate the effect of five factors on the release profile. The factors were the percentage of polymers P1 (hydrophobic cellulose ether type) and P2 (a mono phthalic acid ester type) as well as the spray rate, atomization pressure, substrate type, and temperature. She saw no practical difference between the dissolution release profiles for the first four trials, and the team was no closer to the desired target profile. After contemplating the issue, she decided to switch the order of application of the two polymers. They applied Polymer P2 first, followed by Polymer P1. The release profiles changed significantly and were close to the target. The team had to terminate the trials because they had been instructed to manufacture clinical trial materials for a relative bioavailability study in humans. If the relative bioavailability studies met the study criteria the team would develop the process and product for registration studies.

- Evelyn, the process engineer, and Andrei, the formulator, had to deposit a drug substance on the tablet's surface for an early Phase 1 study. The placebo tablet design onto which they would deposit the drug substance was fixed. After much deliberation, Evelyn and Andrei decided to spray a coating suspension with micronized drug substance onto the tablet surface. The target was 4.50 mg ± 0.45 mg per tablet with a less than 6% RSD. Chester, the statistician, designed a 2^{4-1} design in four blocks since only two trials could be completed in a day. They conducted four trials over two days, after which they were informed the drug substance had to be reallocated for other critical nonclinical studies for the investigational new drug (IND) filing. The management asked if Evelyn and Andrei had enough data to manufacture clinical trial material for an IND study. The alternative was to continue with the nonclinical studies, wait for additional drug substances, and continue the manufacturing studies later. This would delay the regulatory filing and start of the clinical study, which was critical for the company. The four trials gave the data below:

Trials	Block	Duration of spray	Pan speed	Pan load	Atomization pressure	Uniformity of dosage units, mg		
						Average	SD	RSD
8	1	–	–	–	–	3.70	0.27	7.30
1	1	+	+	+	+	3.82	0.24	6.28
2	2	+	–	–	+	4.63	0.17	3.67
7	2	–	+	+	–	3.91	0.21	5.37

SD: Standard deviation; RSD: Relative standard deviation

An experimental design approach can solve the problem or identify a winner. In this case, Evelyn and Andrei acknowledged they did not understand which factors influenced the uniformity of dosage units but decided the risk was low in manufacturing clinical trial supplies using the conditions from Trial 2:

- At this early stage of development, it was more important to know if the drug was safe and effective in a patient population than to completely understand the manufacturing process.
- If the clinical supplies manufacturing campaign failed, they would develop the process as planned here, and the program would be delayed.
- They reviewed the records from the four trials and identified interim measurements and additional controls to lower the risk of failure.

Enforce data quality

Experimenters are aware of Twyman's law as cited by Andrew Ehrenberg that any figure that looks interesting or different is likely to be wrong. We are all too familiar with mismanaged experiments, missing observations, and suspect observations, and enforcing data quality is good practice.

Check for suspect values in the data.

A normal plot of the effects is a diagnostic tool that alerts the investigator to the possibility of a suspect value. Lee, the polymer chemist at On3alpha, experienced this in developing the laboratory synthesis for a hydrophilic polymer, OA391. On3alpha had decided to evaluate the scale-up feasibility.

Lee discussed the 11 factors that could be important during the scale-up process (Table 10.1) with Florence, the statistician. Florence suggested a 12-trial Plackett-Burman design (Table 10.2). Lee wanted to study the raw material from two suppliers. Florence agreed they could include it as a factor. Still, she cautioned Lee that any inference drawn from this study would be tentative because they would use a single and not multiple lots from each supplier. They would have to reevaluate the suppliers in the future. Lee and Andre, the engineer, completed the pilot plant trials. Hiroshi, the analytical chemist, measured the percentage of conversion (P) and color index (W) for two responses. Maximizing P was essential to On3alpha, and maximizing C was necessary to On3alpha's customers.

Table 10.1: The factors evaluated in the scale-up synthesis of OA391 hydrophilic polymer.

Factor	Description	Units
A	pH	
B	Temperature	°C
C	Catalyst feed rate	g/min
D	Stirring rate	rpm
E	Stirrer type	
F	Pre-treatment	
G	Catalyst addition time	min
H	Catalyst concentration	%
I	Reaction time	min
J	Raw material supplier	
K	Drying time	min
Response		
P	Conversion (Target >55%)	%
W	Color index (Target >30)	unitless

Table 10.2: A 12-trial Placket Burman design to study the scale-up synthesis for OA391 hydrophilic polymer.

Trial	Order	A	B	C	D	E	F	G	H	I	J	K	P	W
1	5	+	+	–	+	+	+	–	–	–	+	–	60	35
2	7	+	–	+	+	+	–	–	–	+	–	+	60	31
3	8	–	+	+	+	–	–	–	+	–	+	+	43	39
4	10	+	+	+	–	–	–	+	–	+	+	–	60	32
5	4	+	+	–	–	–	+	–	+	+	–	+	48	39
6	2	+	–	–	–	+	–	+	+	–	+	+	45	36
7	9	–	–	–	+	–	+	+	–	+	+	+	60	22
8	6	–	–	+	–	+	+	–	+	+	+	–	44	25
9	11	–	+	–	+	+	–	+	+	+	–	–	47	37
10	12	+	–	+	+	–	+	+	+	–	–	–	54	32
11	3	–	+	+	–	+	+	+	–	–	–	+	58	29
12	1	–	–	–	–	–	–	–	–	–	–	–	59	27

The normal plot for response P (percentage of conversion) in Figure 10.1 shows the catalyst concentration, H, seems to be the only significant effect. However, we also notice a peculiarity in the normal plot of the effects. The nonsignificant effects seem to split into two groups with a gap around zero, as shown in the second plot in Figure 10.1. This could be because, in the calculations of these insignificant factors, a constant amount is added (or subtracted) from the effect calculation, indicating possible suspect value(s) or typo(s) in the recorded responses. To investigate this, we can consider the signs of the insignificant effects, as shown in the bottom row of Table 10.3. We can see these signs match Experiment 10. Upon further examining the details for Trial 10, Lee and Andre found precisely 1.5 times the low level of the catalyst concentration had been added, which gave the value of 54. This aligned with calculations, and Lee did not repeat the trial.

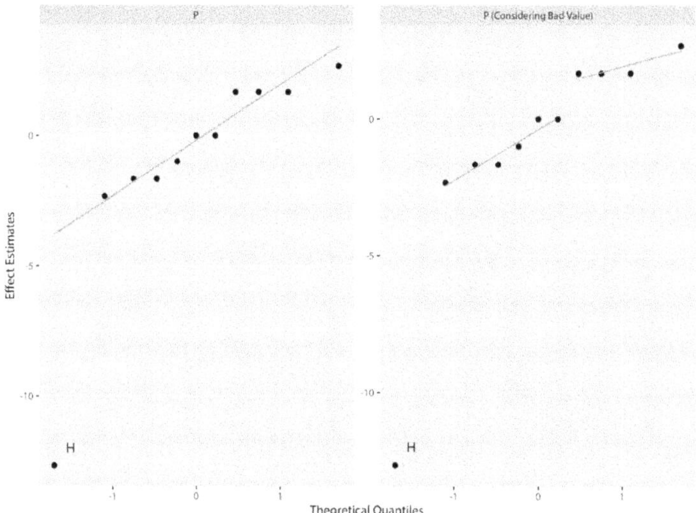

Figure 10.1: The normal plot of the effects for percentage of conversion P from the 12-trial Placket Burman design to study the scale-up synthesis for OA391 hydrophilic polymer. The normal plot on the left shows the catalyst concentration may be affecting P. The normal plot on the right shows the nonsignificant effects split into two groups, indicating a suspect value in the percentage of conversion P.

Table 10.3: Identifying the trial with the suspect value (Trial 10) for percent conversion P by matching the signs of the effects to the coded factor settings in the trial.

Trial	A	B	C	D	E	F	G	H	I	J	K	P
1	+	+	−	+	+	+	−	−	−	+	−	60
2	+	−	+	+	+	−	−	−	+	−	+	60
3	−	+	+	+	−	−	−	+	−	+	+	43
4	+	+	+	−	−	−	+	−	+	+	−	60
5	+	+	−	−	−	+	−	+	+	−	+	48
6	+	−	−	−	+	−	+	+	−	+	+	45
7	−	−	−	+	−	+	+	−	+	+	+	60
8	−	−	+	−	+	+	−	+	+	+	−	44
9	−	+	−	+	+	−	+	+	+	−	−	47
10	+	−	+	+	−	+	+	+	−	−	−	54
11	−	+	+	−	+	+	+	−	−	−	+	58
12	−	−	−	−	−	−	−	−	−	−	−	59
Effect Estimates	2.7	−1	0	1.7	−1.7	1.7	1.7	−12.7	0	−2.3	−1.7	
Signs of Insignificant Effects	+	−		+	−	+	+			−	−	

The normal plot of the effects for response W in Figure 10.2 does not show any significant effects. Like the normal plot of the effects for response P, the effects for response W are split into two groups with different slopes, as shown in the second plot in Figure 10.2. Upon examining the records, Hiroshi found a transcription error for Trial 11. The instrument printout and the notebook recording were both 39, but the analyst had transcribed it as 29 and sent the wrong data to the team.

When the response W for Trial 11 was changed to 39, temperature B seems to be significant, as shown in Figure 10.3. However, there still seems to be a separation between the groups of effect estimates. As shown in Table 10.4. identifying the trial with the suspect value is not straightforward, as the signs of the nonsignificant effects do not match any of the trials. In the right-hand plot of Figure 10.3, we cannot separate the plus and minus sign effects as we did in Figure 10.10 and Table 10.3. The responses were split based on the gap seen in Figure 10.3. The experimenters were concerned the response W of Trial 6 was suspect. This speculation was not supported after examining the measurement records and the experimental datasheets. However, since the project goals were satisfied, Lee planned confirmatory trials to produce the product for evaluation by On3alpha customers.

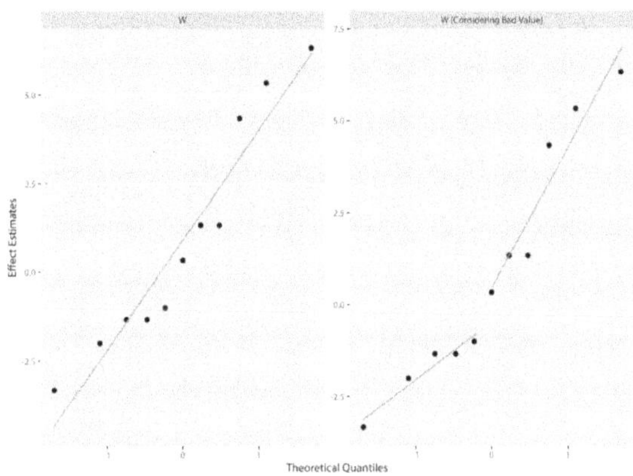

Figure 10.2: The normal plot of the effects for color index W from the 12-trial Placket Burman design to study the scale-up synthesis for OA391 hydrophilic polymer. The plot on the left shows no factor significantly affecting W. The normal plot on the right shows the nonsignificant effects split into two groups, indicating a suspect value in color index W.

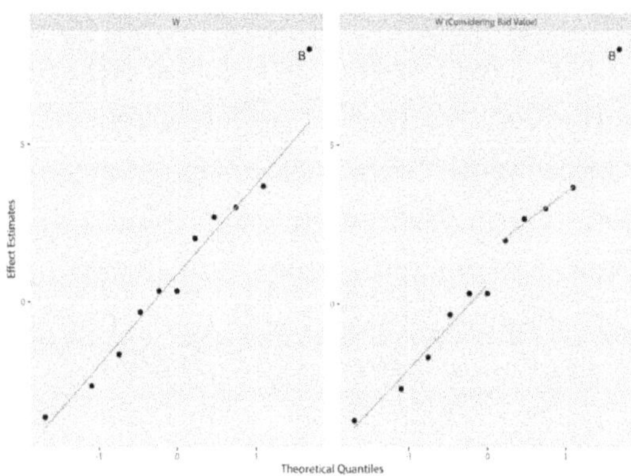

Figure 10.3: The normal plot of the effects for color index W from the 12-trial Placket Burman design to study the scale-up synthesis for OA391 hydrophilic polymer after changing the response for Trial 11 from 29 to 39. The normal plot on the right shows the temperature B may be affecting W. The normal plot on the right shows the nonsignificant effects split into two groups, indicating another suspect value in color index W.

Table 10.4: Identifying the trial with the suspect value for color index W after correcting the response of Trial 11.

Trial	A	B	C	D	E	F	G	H	I	J	K	W
1	+	+	−	+	+	+	−	−	−	+	−	35
2	+	−	+	+	+	−	−	−	+	−	+	31
3	−	+	+	+	−	−	−	+	−	+	+	39
4	+	+	+	−	−	−	+	−	+	+	−	32
5	+	+	−	−	−	+	−	+	+	−	+	39
6	+	−	−	−	+	−	+	+	−	+	+	36
7	−	−	−	+	−	+	+	−	+	+	+	22
8	−	−	+	−	+	+	−	+	+	+	−	25
9	−	+	−	+	+	−	+	+	+	−	−	37
10	+	−	+	+	−	+	+	+	−	−	−	32
11	−	+	+	−	+	+	+	−	−	−	+	39
12	−	−	−	−	−	−	−	−	−	−	−	27
Effect Estimates	2.6	8	0.3	−0.3	2	−1.7	0.3	3.7	−3.7	−2.7	3	
Signs of Insignificant Effects	+		+	−	+	−	+	+	−	−	+	

Lee ran three scale-up batches using the conclusions from the 12-trial Placket Burman design and manufactured the product for evaluation by On3alpha customers (Table 10.5.) A low-catalyst concentration (H) was used to maximize percentage of conversion P. A high temperature (B) was maintained to maximize color index W. All other factors were set at a convenient level based on cycle time. A residual analysis can help with the identification of suspect values. For further details on this we refer the readers to Box, Hunter, and Hunter (2005).

Table 10.5: Data from the three scale-up batches of OA391 hydrophilic polymer to confirm the 12-trial Placket Burman design conclusions.

Factor	Description	Units	Setting	P	W
A	pH	H^+	–	59	32
B	Temperature	°C	+	60	35
C	Catalyst feed rate	g/min	+	59	34
D	Stirring rate	rpm	–		
E	Stirrer type	1 or 2	–		
F	Pre treatment	Y or N	–		
G	Catalyst addition time	min	+		
H	Catalyst concentration	%	–		
I	Reaction time	min	–		
I	Reaction time	min	–		
J	Raw material supplier	A or B	–		
K	Drying time	min	–		

P: Percent conversion
W: Color index

But what about missing values?

Francoise had designed eight trials to evaluate three factors in a spray-drying operation. The aim was to identify the process parameters that would maximize the bulk density of the spray-dried dispersion. The resources, including the raw materials and the pilot plant, were available for eight trials in 8 days. Unfortunately, on the last day, one of the seals in the pressure pump used to vary the feed rate failed, and despite the efforts of the maintenance department, the pump could not be repaired in time, and a backup pump was not available. Francoise reviewed the batch records from the previous trials and confirmed there were no issues in maintaining the pump pressure and other parameters. The pilot plant personnel investigated why they had failed to identify the potential seal failure. They revised the early warning systems for impending equipment malfunction, setup, and maintenance approaches. However, the pilot plant had other projects that could not be delayed, and Francoise had to decide her next steps based on the seven trials. Table 10.6 shows the trials with the missing data.

Table 10.6: A 2^3 design to evaluate the effect of outlet temperature, feed pressure, and nozzle size on the bulk density of a spray-dried dispersion.

Trial	Order	Outlet Temperature °C (A)	Feed Pressure Bar (B)	Nozzle Size mm (C)	ABC	Bulk Density g/cc
1	5	–	–	–	–	0.194
2	1	+	–	–	+	0.136
3	8	–	+	–	+	No data
4	6	+	+	–	–	0.116
5	4	–	–	+	+	0.190
6	3	+	–	+	–	0.141
7	2	–	+	+	–	0.169
8	7	+	+	+	+	0.123

Wright, the statistician, showed Francoise two ways to deal with the missing data:

1. Ignore Trial 3 and perform the regression analysis for the seven available experiments. Of course, that would mean that we would no longer enjoy the excellent properties

of the original design as in the case of orthogonality or balance; for example, in the seven experiments, the temperature would be evaluated four times at the high level and only three times at the low level.

2. To recover the missing data, replace it with a "good" guess of what it could be. The most straightforward approach is to assume that a high-order interaction, e.g., ABC in this case, is, in fact, negligible and hence set to 0. We can then back-calculate the missing response for the third trial so that ABC will exactly be equal to 0. In this example, this gives 0.171 g/cc. Once we have this substitute for the missing response, we can then analyze the data as we would for a standard 2^3 design. (Using the ABC column signs in Table 10.6 and writing x for the data in Row 3 we get $- 0.194 + 0.136 + x - 0.116 + 0.190 - 0.141 - 0.169 + 0.123 = 0$, and $x = 0.171$.)
3. A normal plot using 0.171 as the data for the missing value would indicate the outlet temperature A and feed pressure B could be significant. The 2^3 design in Table 10.6 becomes a replicated 2^2 design for factors A and B. In the next series of trials, Francoise maintained a low outlet temperature A and a low feed pressure B to maximize the bulk density of the spray-dried dispersion. She chose the smaller nozzle size because it was a standard inventory item.

If we bungle or mismanage an experimental trial in an experimental design matrix, we can use the simple procedure outlined here to plug in a fitted value and carry out the analysis. But we should remember a technique is only as good as the assumptions underlying it. So, we seek to choose the higher-order interaction we think is likely to have a small effect. It is also important to answer the questions, "Why was the experiment mismanaged?" and "Why is the observation missing?"

Look beyond the numbers. Avoid the single-number trap.

Miriam, the statistician at Mu6, came across a management summary of a process: "The manufacturing process has a Cpk of 1.82, with a specification of 63.3–70.0%. This means that this process will produce approximately 40 nonconforming products out of a million products and is considered capable. Drug product assay values used to calculate the Cpk were between 64.7% and 67.2%, as shown in Table 1." The report further discussed how the management's quality enhancement policies were effective and urged continuous improvement. Table 10.7 shows the data.

Table 10.7: Percentage of assay values for 42 drug product lots manufactured at a commercial facility.

Batch	% Assay	Batch	% Assay	Batch	% Assay	Batch	% Assay
1	66.9	12	65.1	23	66.3	34	65.8
2	66.3	13	66.6	24	67.1	35	66.0
3	66.2	14	67.2	25	66.5	36	65.9
4	67.0	15	67.1	26	65.9	37	64.7
5	66.2	16	67.2	27	65.8	38	65.2
6	67.2	17	66.5	28	65.7	39	65.8
7	65.9	18	66.5	29	65.1	40	64.7
8	65.8	19	66.3	30	65.5	41	65.9
9	66.1	20	67.1	31	65.5	42	64.7
10	66.5	21	66.5	32	66.3		
11	66.5	22	66.9	33	65.3		

Miriam was curious and decided to visualize the voice of the process by simply plotting the data in time (Figure 10.4).

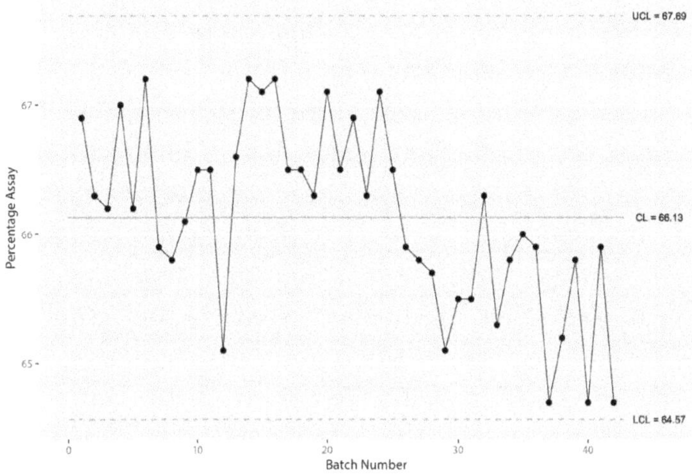

Figure 10.4: Individual control chart for the drug product assay values (using first 25 batches).

She also decided to draw a line representing the average of the responses for all batches to use as a benchmark for the central tendency of the process. She further decided to calculate the standard deviation based on the moving range of the first 25 individual assay values and draw two additional lines that are three standard deviations above and below the average line to represent the natural variation in the process. If the responses are normally distributed, we can show that approximately three out of 1,000 responses would be outside the band represented by these lines. In this format, the figure is a control chart used to determine whether a process operates as expected under random changes or shows excessive variation due to a specific cause. The signals in the control chart in Figure 10.4 include eight successive values falling on the same side of the centerline after Batch 12 and a downward shift after Batch 25. Miriam concluded the manufacturing process was not stable. This is not obvious from the single number, Cpk, used to summarize the data. Please note that Miriam was careful not to add more lines representing the specification limits as she investigated the natural variation in the data.

To compare this variation to the specification limits, as in the case of Cpk, Miriam decided to plot the histogram of the data, which shows the process is not centered within the specification limits. The available elbow room is less at the lower specification than that at the higher specification. The process is off-center but has not yet produced nonconforming products.

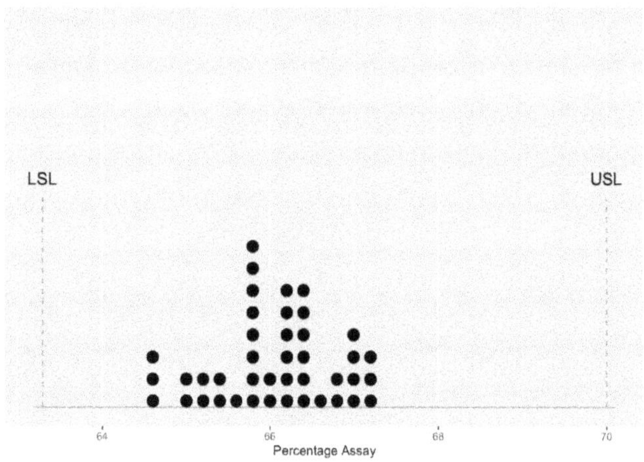

Figure 10.5: Histogram for the individual drug product assay values.

Amidst the rapidly changing, highly fragmented, frequently interrupted, and often ambiguous workday characterized by time constraints, it is easy to feel that errors in data interpretation do not matter, so long as one is producing products conforming to the specification. But the process will eventually drift if unattended and produce nonconforming products, creating crises or a whack-a-mole approach to preventing them.

When one has the luxury of time, a better approach is to make the process stable and centered using process knowledge, the control chart, and the histogram. While a single number reduces the complexity of information, it is often a trap that does not allow us to visualize the data and understand how the process behaves over time. One way to reduce the narrow view of a single number is to ask, "What data was used to calculate the single number?" and "Does the data show a trend, anomalies, or patterns even if the product meets specifications?"

A good solution now is usually better than a perfect one later.

This book suffers from an over reliance on two-level factorial designs, and, as Maslow's hammer suggests, everything appears as a nail if all you have is a hammer. The two-level factorial plans are the workhorse for experimentation because they are flexible and adaptable to various situations. And in this case they offer a good solution rather than a perfect one.

While we should take advantage of advances in experimental design, we should not lose sight of the bigger picture in product development. Could experimenters choose a plan theoretically tailored to their goal and circumstances? Yes. Could they do an analysis yielding better estimates? Perhaps. Is there a tailored approach for their situation? Could be. We could do better in theory. But in practice, the costs of doing better may be so high that a good solution is actually better than a perfect one. Without a crystal ball, it isn't easy to get things right. Counterintuitive as it seems, the best solution is often the simplest—and most straightforward to use—and not the best in theory. Product developers usually avoid complexity where simplicity has much greater explanatory power. We mine the diamonds of simplicity before turning to the rhinestones of complexity. Besides, the sequential approach allows one to course-correct as the investigation advances. An experimental design must be a means to learn and not an end for practitioners.

Anchor your experimental strategy to realities on the ground.

Any experimental effort involves risks, which few will be willing to take unless there is organizational support. Experimenters struggle with decisions, especially when the awkward realities on the floor, cost, team dynamics, the need to show progress, and careers are involved. Other factors that could influence the experimental strategy include work relationships and the level of knowledge.

The sequential approach will not avoid the remorse expressed by Helmholtz as quoted in Chapter 1. When an experimenter looks back at the investigation or the development, they may wonder why they did not arrive at a solution or develop a product sooner.

Use design thinking to strategize resources.

When an experimenter starts thinking in 4, 6, 8, 12, and 16 trials, they can estimate the resources they will need more efficiently, including raw material, laboratories, manufacturing units, equipment use, time, and money. For example, if they need eight experiments to develop a process and each trial is estimated at $8,000 to $11,000 to complete and test, they will need $64,000 to $88,000. Experience teaches us to multiply the budget by 1.3 to 3.0 because of the uncertainty in development. Similarly, timelines are estimated by considering the sequential and parallel tasks needed for the trials and working with project managers, operations, and others to outline the project plan.

Experimental design is not just a hypothesis-testing tool.

When we fail to acknowledge the iterative and recursive nature of experimentation and data analysis, forget the difference between statistical and practical significance, and do not interact with the data and analysis using subject matter knowledge, we fail to learn effectively, use experimental design as a p-value provider, and miss the opportunity to develop a product from exploration to manufacturing systematically.

We do not use p-values mechanically to decide on the effects to act on and those to ignore. We interact with statistical information about the size of the effect and its possible error with our subject matter knowledge.

All that is gold does not glitter. Not all those who wander are lost.

—J. R. R. Tolkien

We have in this book often considered experimentation as means for learning and discovery and frequently promoted sequential experimentation that can easily make the experimenter wander onto an unexplored path. We would also like to use this quote from Tolkien to emphasize that this certainly does not imply that the experimenter is lost. She has embarked on a journey where systematic trials will most likely lead to success. The first part of the quote, "All that is gold does not glitter," can imply that discoveries can be made in unexpected twists and turns along our sequential experimental design journey.

One last thing

The sequential experimental design approach with subject matter knowledge may not lead you toward your goals in a smoothly rising ramp or guarantee a solution. Still, it can help you self-correct toward your goal, provide a satisfactory resolution, and use resources sensibly by mapping a path toward the goals.

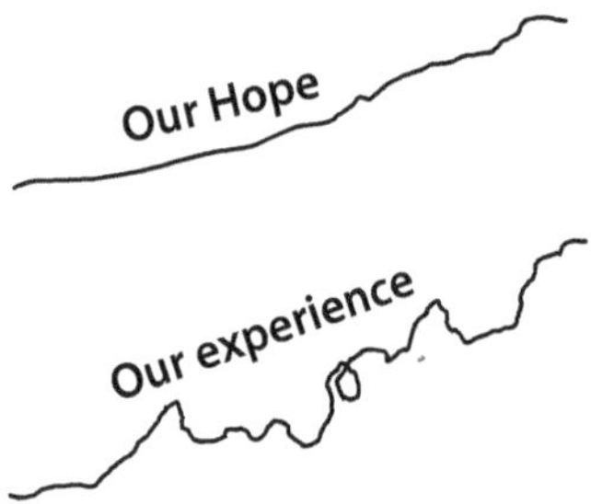

As he describes in his bestselling 1998 memoir *Rocket Boys* (and as the movie based on his book, *October Sky,* depicted), NASA engineer Homer Hickam, Jr., started designing and building rockets as a boy. He was 14 years old in 1957 when the Sputnik launch occurred, and watching it on television inspired him. He began experimenting with a flashlight tube and a model airplane body as a casing in his backyard. Flash powder from old cherry bombs fueled the rocket. Unfortunately, the explosion destroyed a fence. Undaunted, Hickam enlisted five friends, and the so-called "Rocket Boys" found community support to design, develop, and launch the rockets they made. The community's response in advice, encouragement, space, materials, money, and other aids led to the launch of 35 experimental rockets by 1960. The Rocket Boys won the National Science Fair gold medal for their work.

Hickam's memoir outlines a process of trial-and-error experimentation that relied on ingenuity, perseverance, and subject matter knowledge. But combining statistical experimental design, creativity, persistence, and subject matter knowledge can ease the slow and laborious ascent to a solution.

Ideas develop step by step, and the sequential experimental design strategy matches this. When looking at empirical data, we often ask, how do the factors affect the response? Why are the factors doing what they do?[1] And what to do next? We build experiments in sequence using what we know and have learned from the previous experiments. The length of time developing a pharmaceutical product takes masks the iterative nature of experimentation. We see the broader picture when we step back and write down what occurred over the years when filing the new drug application and getting it approved for a broader patient population. Product development is cumulative and progressive.

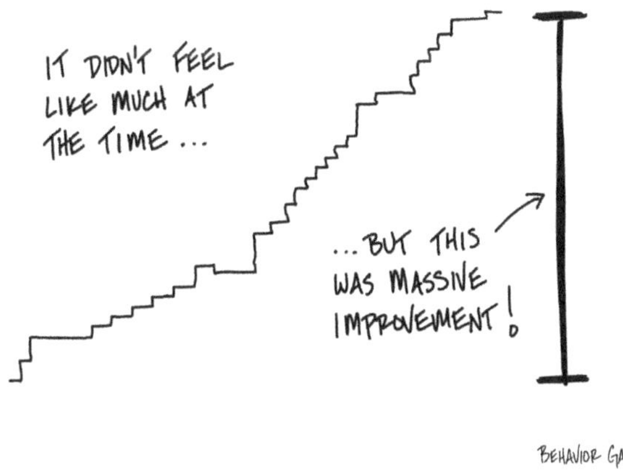

IT DIDN'T FEEL LIKE MUCH AT THE TIME ...
... BUT THIS WAS MASSIVE IMPROVEMENT!
BEHAVIOR GAP

1 We have not reasoned the data in-depth from a technical subject matter view because it is outside the scope of this book.

NOTES

Box, G.E.P. (2006). *Improving Almost Anything*. New York: Wiley.

Daniel, C. (1994). Factorial One-Factor-at-a-Time Experiments. *The American Statistician* 48 (2): 132–135.

Ehrenberg, A.S.C. (1975). *Data Reduction*. New York: Wiley.

England, P. C., Molnar, P., and Richter, F.M. (2007). Kelvin, Perry and the Age of the Earth. *American Scientist* 95 (4): 342–349.

Hickam, H. (1998). *Rocket Boys*. New York: Random House Publishing.

Wheeler, D. and Chambers, D. (2010). *Understanding Statistical Process Control*. Third edition. Knoxville, TN: SPC Press.

The procedure for the individual control chart:

Calculate the average ($\overline{X}$) of the time-ordered data set.
Calculate the moving range (MR) by computing the absolute difference. between successive values in the data set.
Calculate the average moving range ($\overline{MR}$).
Calculate the lower and upper control limits: $\overline{X} \pm (2.66 \times \overline{MR})$.

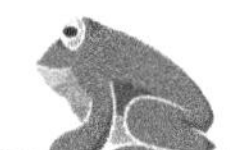

The copyright holders of specific illustrations are credited: Chapter 2: Portfolio design by Carl Richards, Behavior Gap. Chapter 3: Current reality by Carl Richards, Behavior Gap. Chapter 4: Fast by Amy Hwang, Conde Nast TCB-147868. Chapter 9: Problems by Frank Cotham, Cartoon Stock CC32988. Chapter 10: Hindsight, Foresight by Tim Cordell, Cartoon Stock CS467780. Ankles by Amy Hwang, Conde Nast TCB-146898. Incremental change by Carl Richards, Behavior Gap. Every effort has been made to trace or contact all copyright holders. Any inadvertent omissions will be rectified at the earliest opportunity.

Credits: Kate Epstein and Elizabeth Crooks for editorial assistance, Smitha Pisharam for certain illustrations, and Anna Staskiewicz for sketchnotes.

This Is Experimenting

We wish to show you
Roughly how
to experiment.

Know some factors,
J,I,T — Design begins
Get some levels two or three
Take a -
low down
Take a +
high up,
Take a 0
center city,
Measure a response
one that counts
Use a factorial
Rothamstead born.
Now you are designing
your experiments.
If you experience turbulence,
Take our tip
That's part of the fun.

In Berkeley,
mathematistry is all
optimal hot.
Daniel on the Taber
Beat one at a time.
Split-plot plans are
good, good, good.
In software today,
The search is for
alias optimals.
But through it all
at all the stages
Keep in mind
the environment and
the time.

From the floor
Up to the offices,
Think design
From the labs
Out to the factory,
Design is king.

www.ingramcontent.com/pod-product-compliance
Lightning Source LLC
Chambersburg PA
CBHW040932210326
41597CB00030B/5272

* 9 7 9 8 9 8 7 1 0 8 6 1 1 *